Foot & Ankle Innovations in Latin America

Guest Editors

CRISTIAN ORTIZ, MD
EMILIO WAGNER, MD

FOOT AND ANKLE CLINICS

www.foot.theclinics.com

Consulting Editor
MARK S. MYERSON, MD

September 2012 • Volume 17 • Number 3

SAUNDERS an imprint of ELSEVIER, Inc.

W.B. SAUNDERS COMPANY
A Division of Elsevier Inc.

1600 John F. Kennedy Blvd. ● Suite 1800 ● Philadelphia, PA 19103-2899

http://www.theclinics.com

FOOT AND ANKLE CLINICS Volume 17, Number 3
September 2012 ISSN 1083-7515, ISBN-13: 978-1-4557-4952-2

Editor: David Parsons
Developmental Editor: Teia Stone

Foot and Ankle Clinics (ISSN 1083-7515) is published quarterly by Elsevier, Inc., 360 Park Avenue South, New York, NY 10010-1710. Months of issue are March, June, September, and December. Periodicals postage paid at New York, NY, and additional mailing offices. Subscription price per year is $295.00 (US individuals), $386.00 (US institutions), $146.00 (US students), $336.00 (Canadian individuals), $456.00 (Canadian institutions), $201.00 (Canadian students), $433.00 (foreign individuals), $456.00 (foreign institutions), and $201.00 (foreign students). To receive student/resident rate, orders must be accompanied by name of affiliated institution, date of term, and the *signature* of program/residency coordinator on institution letterhead. Orders will be billed at individual rate until proof of status is received. Foreign air speed delivery is included in all *Clinics* subscription prices. All prices are subject to change without notice. **POSTMASTER:** Send address changes to *Foot and Ankle Clinics*, Elsevier Health Sciences Division, Subscription Customer Service, 3251 Riverport Lane, Maryland Heights, MO 63043. **Customer Service: 1-800-654-2452 (US and Canada). From outside of the United States and Canada, call 314-447-8871. Fax: 314-447-8029. E-mail: JournalsCustomerService-usa@ elsevier.com (for print support); JournalsOnlineSupport-usa@elsevier.com (for online support).**

Reprints. For copies of 100 or more, of articles in this publication, please contact the Commercial Reprints Department, Elsevier Inc., 360 Park Avenue South, New York, NY 10010-1710. Tel.: 212-633-3812; Fax: 212-462-1935; E-mail: reprints@elsevier.com.

Printed and bound by CPI Group (UK) Ltd, Croydon, CR0 4YY

Transferred to Digital Print 2012

Contributors

CONSULTING EDITOR

MARK S. MYERSON, MD
Director, Institute for Foot and Ankle Reconstruction at Mercy, Mercy Medical Center, Baltimore, Maryland

GUEST EDITORS

CRISTIAN ORTIZ, MD
Chief, Foot and Ankle Service; Vice-President, Chilean Orthopedic and Traumatology Society; Associate Professor, Universidad del Desarrollo; Clinica Alemana, Vitacura, Santiago, Chile

EMILIO WAGNER, MD
Chief, Foot and Ankle Service Hospital Padre Hurtado; Staff Member, Foot and Ankle Service; Associate Professor, Universidad del Desarrollo; Clinica Alemana, Vitacura, Santiago, Chile

AUTHORS

GUILLERMO ARRONDO, MD
Staff of Foot and Ankle Servicie at Institute Dupuytren, Buenos Aires, Argentina

JUAN BERNARDO GERSTNER GARCES, MD
Centro Medico Imbanaco, Instituto de Enfermedades Osteoarticulars, Cali, Colombia

JOSE CARLOS COHEN, MD
Chief, Foot and Ankle Service, Department of Orthopaedic Surgery, Federal University Hospital of Rio de Janeiro-UFRJ, Rio de Janeiro, Brazil

YEARSON DIEGO, MD
Staff of Foot and Ankle Servicie at Institute Dupuytren, Buenos Aires, Argentina

ELIFAZ DE FREITAS CABRAL, MD
Consultant Orthopaedic Surgeon, Health State Department of Brazil for Rehabilitation and Prevention in Hansen's Disease; Associate Professor of Medicine, Faculdade Integrada São Lucas, Rondônia, Brazil

JOÃO L. ELLERA GOMES, MD, PhD
Associated Professor, Department of Orthopaedic and Traumatoly, HCPA, FAMED-UFRGS, Universidade Federal do Rio Grande do Sul, Porto Alegre, Brazil

SANTIAGO ESLAVA, MD
Staff of Foot and Ankle Servicie at Institute Dupuytren, Buenos Aires, Argentina

ANAIN FEDERICO, MD
Staff of Foot and Ankle Servicie at Institute Dupuytren, Buenos Aires, Argentina

C. SERGIO FERNÁNDEZ, MD
Chief, Foot & Ankle, Orthopedics and Traumatology Department, Clínica Santa María; Professor Orthopedic & Traumatology, Universidad de Los Andes, Santiago, Chile

JOSÉ FELIPE MARION ALLOZA, MD
Post Graduation in Orthopaedics/Assistant at the Foot and Ankle Clinic and Sports Medicine Clinic, Federal University of São Paulo-UNIFESP, Escola Paulista de Medicina, São Paulo, Brazil

GERMAN JOANNAS, MD
Staff of Foot and Ankle Servicie at Institute Dupuytren, Buenos Aires, Argentina

CESAR KHAZEN, MD
Unidad de Pié y Tobillo, Hospital de Clínicas Caracas, Caracas, Venezuela

GABRIEL KHAZEN, MD
Unidad de Pié y Tobillo, Hospital de Clínicas Caracas, Caracas, Venezuela

A. MIGUES, MD
Institute of Orthopaedics "Carlos E. Ottolenghi," Italian Hospital of Buenos Aires, Buenos Aires, Argentina

ALBERTO MACKLIN VADELL, MD
EPTP-Buenos Aires, Sanatorio Mater Dei, Buenos Aires, Argentina

CAIO NERY, MD
Associate Professor, Head of the Orthopaedic Discipline, Federal University of São Paulo-UNIFESP, Escola Paulista de Medicina, São Paulo, Brazil

DANIEL NIÑO GOMEZ, MD
Chief of Foot and Ankle Servicie at Institute Dupuytren, Buenos Aires, Argentina

CRISTIAN ORTIZ, MD
Chief, Foot and Ankle Service; Vice-President, Chilean Orthopedic and Traumatology Society; Associate Professor, Universidad del Desarrollo; Clinica Alemana, Vitacura, Santiago, Chile

MARCELA PERATTA, MD
EPTP-Buenos Aires, Sanatorio Mater Dei, Buenos Aires, Argentina

CIBELE RÉSSIO, MD
Post Grade in Orthopaedics/Assistant at the Foot and Ankle Clinic, Federal University of São Paulo-UNIFESP, Escola Paulista de Medicina, São Paulo, Brazil

JOSÉ A.V. SANHUDO, MD
Doctor's Degree HCPA, FAMED-UFRGS, Orthopaedic and Traumatology Service, Mãe de Deus Hospital, Porto Alegre, Brazil

GASTÓN SLULLITEL, MD
Institute of Orthopadics "Dr. Jaime Slullitel", Pueyrredon, Santa Fe, Argentina

EMILIO WAGNER, MD
Chief, Foot and Ankle Service Hospital Padre Hurtado; Staff Member, Foot and Ankle Service; Associate Professor, Universidad del Desarrollo; Clinica Alemana, Vitacura, Santiago, Chile

Contents

Chronic ankle instability is one of the most common problems in foot and ankle surgery, for which anatomic reconstruction is the procedure of choice despite presenting possible complications. Nonanatomic techniques can lead to permanent changes in ankle kinematics. To minimize surgical exposure while obtaining results as good as for open procedures, and in hopes of decreasing complications, an arthroscopic approach has been developed by the author. The results confirm a simple, effective, and efficient technique for reconstruction of the ankle ligament, with a low complication rate, which does not close the door on anatomic or nonanatomic reconstructions in the future.

Stage I posterior tibial tendon dysfunction (PTTD) is defined as tenosynovitis or tendinitis whereby tendon length remains normal, there is no hindfoot deformity, and diagnosis is basically clinical, characterized by swelling and tenderness posterior to the medial malleolus. This condition is often misdiagnosed as ankle sprain, which delays correct diagnosis and early treatment that may improve symptoms, stop the disease process, and prevent the development of adult acquired flatfoot deformity. Posterior tibial tendoscopic synovectomy is a minimally invasive and effective surgical procedure to treat patients with stage I PTTD.

The treatment of intercuneiform and tarsometatarsal joint fracture dislocations is controversial and many patients develop painful osteoarthritis. This article presents a new surgical technique to reconstruct the ligamentous complex of the region based on the reproduction of its anatomy and isometrics. By making strategic bone tunnels in the cuneiforms and metatarsal bases, the harvesting of the extensor digitorum longus tendon reinforced by an unabsorbable suture gives rise to a neoligament that keeps the joints mobile and flexible. The neoligamentplasty is a valid alternative to the classic treatment of subtle intercuneiform and tarsometatarsal joint lesions.

Plantar plate rupture is a common cause of forefoot pain, multiplanar malalignment, subluxation, or dislocation of the metatarsophalangeal joint

treatment depends on the etiology and severity of the deformity. Operative procedures are divided into joint-preserving techniques (cheilectomy, phalanx, and first metatarsal osteotomies) and joint-sacrificing techniques (arthrodesis, arthroplasty). This article presents a review of the literature and analyzes biomechanical aspects of hallux rigidus, its classification, and etiology, and discusses the available treatment options in the literature along with the authors' own preferred approach.

FOOT AND ANKLE CLINICS

Preface

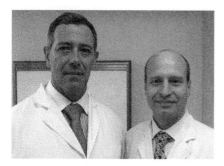

Cristian Ortiz, MD
Emilio Wagner, MD
Guest Editors

It has been a pleasure and a great honor to participate as editors of this issue of *Foot and Ankle Clinics*. In the last few years, South America has been progressively more active in terms of scientific activity. Specifically in foot and ankle, an increasing number of members of our different orthopedic societies have been doing formal training with the world leaders of our subspecialty. This has led South American surgeons to participate in International Societies such as AOFAS and IFFAS as International members, collaborate in different committees, give talks, and also show our scientific work through an increasing number of publications.

The geographic distance that separates our countries from the rest of the world has created a need for us to look for contacts, friendship, and knowledge from all around the world. This relationship has given us a wider spectrum of knowledge than usual and helped us to adapt our surgical knowledge to our local situation. This means that even though in some places in our countries we have ultimate technology and resources available, this is not true everywhere, and sometimes we are forced to use whatever we have and adapt it to our specific population, taking into consideration implant sizes, social network support, insurance requirements, mechanism of injuries, special patient requirements, etc.

We selected for this issue a few specific topics that reflect part of our development projects. For this reason this issue is not just dedicated to one aspect of our subspecialty but more to a compilation of different individual interests. Each one of the authors has done a lot for their own society and for our continental society, FLAME-CIPP (Latin American Federation of Medicine and Surgery of the Leg and Foot), and did a great job working out the final results that are published in this issue. Aspects about Lisfranc fractures, ankle instability, tendon transfers, forefoot disease, and others are discussed and analyzed, taking into consideration current knowledge, local availability of resources, and particularly, social behavior, which many times mandates the management and expected results of our procedures.

Foot Ankle Clin N Am 17 (2012) ix–x
http://dx.doi.org/10.1016/j.fcl.2012.07.003
1083-7515/12/$ – see front matter © 2012 Elsevier Inc. All rights reserved.

This is a great opportunity to thank Elsevier and the consulting editor for the chance given to us to contribute to foot and ankle knowledge. Their friendship and advice were of enormous help in organizing and putting together information coming from six different countries. We also want to thank our teachers and fellowship professor, who provided us with knowledge and ideas to start on this continuous learning process. We hope that this issue reflects part of our effort to increase the scientific development that can be generated from this part of the world, allowing us to get even closer to the rest of the more active scientific producing groups. This with no doubt stimulates us to continue on our learning process and on our teaching duties, helping our residents and fellows to continue improving the quality of research and patient care in this fascinating orthopedic subspecialty.

Cristian Ortiz, MD
Clinica Alemana
Vitacura 5951, Santiago, Chile

Emilio Wagner, MD
Clinica Alemana
Vitacura 5951, Santiago, Chile

E-mail addresses:
caortizm@gmail.com (C. Ortiz)
Emiliowagner@gmail.com (E. Wagner)

Chronic Ankle Instability

Juan Bernardo Gerstner Garces, MD

KEYWORDS

- Ankle instability • Ankle kinematics • Sprain

KEY POINTS

- Among the techniques used to treat chronic ankle instability, the Broström-Gould technique is the most commonly reported, with good to excellent results in the vast majority of cases.
- It is estimated that 10% or more of the consultations in the emergency department are inversion traumas of the ankle, which occur in 1 of every 10,000 people per day.
- A conservative approach is always the first treatment, including anti-inflammatory medications, rehabilitation and proprioception, infiltration with steroids in impingement cases, and use of orthotics, whose true effectiveness is the subject of multiple studies and questions.

INTRODUCTION

Chronic ankle instability is one of the most common problems in foot and ankle surgery, usually presenting after an inversion trauma despite a reliable physical therapy program. The surgeon must rule out several abnormalities that can precipitate this condition such as cavo varus feet, peroneal tendon dislocation, and neuromuscular diseases. Once the diagnosis is made, the most appropriate surgical technique is selected to suit the patient's need according to the level of instability, age, physical activities, and prior surgical procedures. Among the techniques used, the Broström-Gould technique is the most commonly reported, with good to excellent results in the vast majority of cases. Other anatomic techniques, so called when they try to mimic the original location of the ankle ligaments, use different augmentation tissues, such as periosteum, local grafts, or free tendons. Nonanatomic techniques have been used in the past, but currently are not the procedure of choice, as such procedures can lead to permanent changes in ankle kinematics. Anatomic reconstructions also present some complications, such as soft-tissue infections in up to 1.6% and nerve problems in 3.8% of patients. In an effort to minimize surgical exposure while obtaining results comparable with those of open procedures, and in hopes of decreasing complications, an arthroscopic approach has been developed by the author. The results

Centro Medico Imbanaco, Instituto de Enfermedades Osteoarticulars, Carrera 38#5ª-100, Consultorio 233 A, Cali 0002, Colombia
E-mail address: jbgerstner@imbanaco.com.co

Foot Ankle Clin N Am 17 (2012) 389–398
http://dx.doi.org/10.1016/j.fcl.2012.06.001
1083-7515/12/$ – see front matter © 2012 Elsevier Inc. All rights reserved.

foot.theclinics.com

confirm a simple, effective, and efficient technique for reconstruction of the ankle ligament, with a low complication rate, which does not close the door on anatomic or nonanatomic reconstructions in the future.

Ankle sprain is one of the most common lesions associated to sports trauma and in activities of daily life. It is estimated that 10% or more of the consultations in the emergency room (ER) are inversion traumas of the ankle, which occur in 1 of every 10,000 people per day.[1–3] Despite an adequate diagnosis and a protocol of strict management, a group of patients evolve toward chronic instability and residual symptoms of anterolateral impingement and synovitis, and in controlled studies it is estimated that 50% of the cases can evolve with the consequences described.[4,5] The severity of the lesion does not always correspond to the presence of residual symptoms, but does associate with the presence of initial damage of the syndesmosis.[6–8] The lateral region of the ankle contains static and dynamic restrictors of movement. Static restrictors consist of the bony configuration of the ankle including the configuration of the talus, wide in its anterior portion and straight in its subsequent portion; the talofibular mortise and its movement in unison with the talus in dorsal and plantar flexion; and the topography of the distal tibia, which contributes 30% of the restriction to the rotational forces. The dynamic restrictors contribute to the remaining 70% of the constraint of the rotational forces and are chiefly soft tissues, which in their anatomic disposition permit harmonious movements of articulation but also limit the arch of motion of the joint so as not to exceed its functional capacity. These restrictors are the collateral ligaments, the syndesmosis ligaments, and the peroneal tendons. Three clearly defined bands inside the lateral ligaments of the ankle exist: the anterior talofibular ligament (ATF), compromising 68% of the system, and constitutes the main restrictor of the ankle in dorsal to plantar flexion movement. It originates in the anterior ridge of the lateral malleoli, courses in an anteromedial direction, and is inserted in the body of the talus, anterior to the joint facet of the lateral malleoli. Its damage is evaluated by the anterior drawer test, and its severity depends on factors subjectively evaluated by the examiner, but in general it can be classified as of mild, moderate, and severe degree. The fibulocalcaneal ligament (FCL) works synchronically with the ATF, and therefore is rarely injured in isolation. The FCL is involved in 20% of ankle inversion trauma; it originates on the lowest ridge edge of the lateral malleoli and inserts in the lateral surface of the heel bone. Its damage is evaluated by the talar tilt test and is corroborated with a stressed anteroposterior radiograph. The peroneal tendons travel in the retromaleolar lateral zone and are directed through a fibro-osseous tunnel, in an oblique direction, before being inserted in the base of the fifth metatarsal (peroneus brevis), and in the base of the first metatarsal and medial cuneiform (peroneus longus). These tendons work as plantar flexors and evertors, producing 63% of the eversion capacity work and stabilizing the ankle and subtalar joints.

The ligaments of the syndesmosis stabilize the ankle mortise in the movements of dorsal and plantar flexion, while the anteriormost portion (wider) of the talus enters and leaves the mortise. The most inferior portion of the anterior tibiofibular ligament (ligament of Basset) can be compromised in ankle sprains and chronic instability, and can produce hypertrophic scar tissue formation, developing symptoms of impingement in the anterolateral gutter, responsible to a large extent for the residual pain occurring in ankle sprain. The initial damage of the ligaments can be looked for with the compression test, and the external rotation test in the acute setting. After the anterolateral impingement syndrome is established, the examiner finds pain in the anterolateral gutter, and limitation in dorsiflexion caused by pain in the same zone.[9–12]

The classic operative methods for ankle ligament reconstruction have been divided into 2 major groups: anatomic and nonanatomic repairs. Anatomic repairs include reconstruction of the original ligaments by either shortening and reattaching them to the bony surfaces, or augmenting them with surrounding structures to empower the repair. A good example is the classic Broström-Gould repair, which enhances the original ligaments with the extensor retinaculum and has proved to be a strong procedure without sacrificing other anatomic structures. Surgically, a "J" or longitudinal incision is made to gain access to both the anterior and posterior aspects of the fibula; the anterior talofibular ligament and the calcaneal fibular ligament are cut as close to the bone as possible to reattach them in a new groove created to promote a bleeding surface for integration. Peroneal tendons are explored in the posterior aspect of the fibula, and if dislocated they can be repaired at the same time. The extensor retinaculum is finally used as a new layer of tissue on top of the repaired ligaments to reinforce the reconstruction.

Nonanatomic repairs include the use of another structure to accomplish the function of the ligament when it is impossible to repair it directly. Several techniques have been described, including partial or complete tenodesis from the peroneal tendon, Achilles tendon, or tibial tendon; or allografts mimicking the restriction forces of the original ligament such as the Chrisman-Snook, the modified Evans procedure, or the Watson-Jones procedure, to name a few. The modified Chrisman-Snook procedure consists of a repair using the anterior half of the peroneus brevis tendon taken proximally to the tip of the fibula, and then passed through a hole from anterior to posterior, then down to the calcaneus where it is attached with an anchor or a screw with a spiked washer. Generally speaking, nonanatomic repairs are not the preferred reconstruction technique because they impair normal biomechanics and leave residual stiffness.

In an effort to devise a method that could treat ankle instability and the signs and symptoms of impingement and synovitis, with minimum morbidity, ease of reproduction, and good to excellent results within acceptable time limits, arthroscopic treatments have evolved that can address all the aforementioned issues. The advantage of these techniques is that they do not "burn any bridge" for other methods of open and classic stabilization.[13–16]

THE AUTHOR'S PREFERRED METHOD

Continuing the principles of the arthroscopic suture of the medial retinaculum of the knee described by Parisien,[17] the principle of the anatomic reconstruction described by Broström[18] and modified by Gould,[19] the popularization of the arthroscopic surgery of the ankle, and the principle of radiofrequency shrinkage of the joint capsule,[20,21] this method intends to combine all these principles for the stabilization of a lesion of the anterior ATF in unstable ankles in patients with medium and low sport demands without systemic illnesses or deformities in the anatomic axis, who adhere to the protocol of postsurgical rehabilitation.

The surgical technique requires the use of an operating room with a tower for arthroscopy, arthroscopic instruments and lenses of 2.7 and 4.0 mm, shavers and burr instruments for large and small joints, radiofrequency equipment with tips for small joints, and absorbable #2 sutures with cutting needles of sufficient diameter according to the volume of the ankle. The patient is given general or conductive anesthesia, and is placed in a supine position. A pillow under the ipsilateral hip is placed to obtain a mild internal rotation of the extremity and to allow easy access to the lateral gutter. A tourniquet is applied in the manner of an Esmarch elastic band. The superficial peroneal nerve is identified and painted, and the security zone for the placement of the sutures is delimited underneath it (**Fig. 1**).

Initial distension of the joint with saline solution is performed. Through the medial portal the arthroscopy is initiated, proceeding to examine the joint, its gutters, and the joint surface (**Fig. 2**).

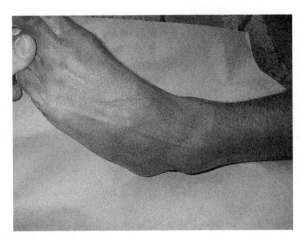

Fig. 1. Superficial peroneal nerve.

The lateral portal is located, and the associated abnormalities previously studied in the context of the instability are corrected (eg, synovitis, impingement syndromes, and osteochondral lesions). The instability is arthroscopically verified, and different points are identified such as the points for anatomic repair, the anterior portion of the fibula, the joint capsule, and the zone of nervous security. A small incision is made in the skin on the anterior fibular edge and a curved needle is introduced, whose emergence in the articulation is controlled by arthroscopy (**Fig. 3**). The needle is then directed anteriorly, taking a great portion of the ligament and the joint capsule, and emerges distally in the skin, thus assuring the inclusion of the extensor retinaculum (**Fig. 4**).

The needle is partially extracted to its union with the suture and is returned in retrograde fashion through the subcutaneous tissue, weaving toward the incision on the anterior fibular edge, where the suture is recovered and subsequently knotted. The procedure is repeated 1 or 2 times more according to the size of the ankle, achieving at a minimum 2 complete sutures (**Fig. 5**).

Arthroscopically the surgeon then proceeds to the shrinkage of the capsule and the ligament (which is partly in the joint) by means of radiofrequency tips in respect of the sutures already placed (**Fig. 6**).

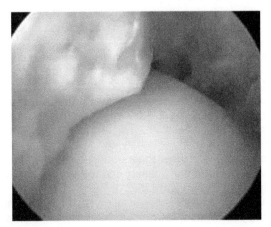

Fig. 2. Lateral gutter.

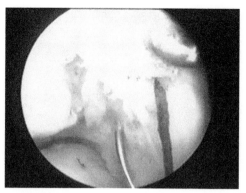

Fig. 3. Needle inside the joint.

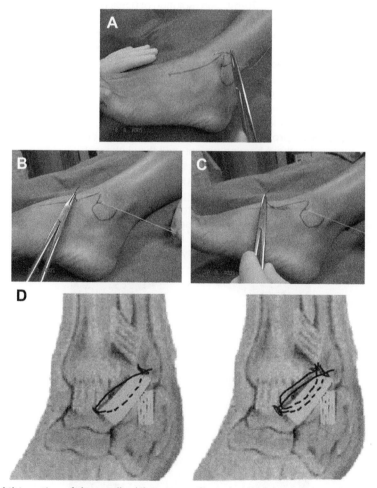

Fig. 4. (*A*) Insertion of the needle. (*B*) First pass through skin. (*C*) Second pass backward. (*D*) Representative diagrams.

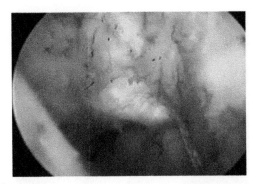

Fig. 5. Sutures in place.

Sutures are knotted in eversion maintained by the assistant, and the stability is verified after knotting.

When closing the portals, a 20-mL pure solution of 0.5% bupivacaine with epinephrine is placed intra-articularly and the ankle is immobilized, with a subsequent placement of plaster on the ankle at 90° with surgical gauzes on the injuries. The patient is handled in an ambulatory way, and is instructed in the use of local ice on the anterior part of the ankle, analgesic medicines, and anti-inflammatory drugs according to the protocol of multimodal analgesia.[22,23]

Patients do not bear weight for a week (except in cases of osteochondral lesions of the talus), at the end of which a cam walker is used for another 3 weeks, before being sent to physical therapy guided by the protocol of Sammarco.[7] In cases of osteochondral lesion, patients are protected for a period of 3 weeks in a plaster, then start range-of-motion exercises without bearing weight until the sixth week.

Alternatively, small (2.0 mm) bony anchors can be used after previous burr preparation of the anterior fibular ridge, placing one in the anterior border of the fibula and another at the point of insertion of the ligament into the talus. The first suture is directed from the inside to the outside of the joint, exiting the skin, then the second suture is redirected through the subcutaneous tissue to the exit point of the first suture, before knotting both (**Figs. 7** and **8**). Anchors are used in cases of good-quality bone stock and based on availability.

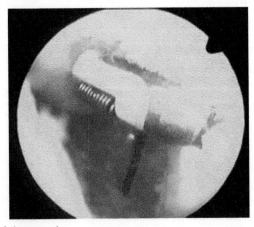

Fig. 6. Shrinkage of the capsule.

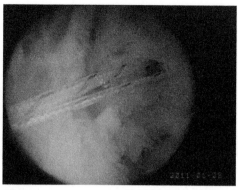

Fig. 7. Anchor is inserted.

Patients with this modification of the original technique were not enrolled in the present study.

RESULTS

Few articles related to arthroscopic repair of the lateral ligaments of the ankle have been published. In 2009 Corte-Real and Moreira[24] described 28 patients treated with an arthroscopic technique of reinforcing the ATF ligament with an anchor placed in the fibula. The average American Orthopedic Foot and Ankle Score (AOFAS)[23] was 85 points, which is excellent considering that the majority were worker-compensation patients. Three had persistent problems (9.6%) of scar tenderness and nerve problems. More recently a case series of 38 patients with 9.8 years of follow-up was described, with good to excellent results in 95% of the cases and an average postoperative AOFAS of 90 points.[25]

In the study by the author's group, 132 patients who were subjected to this particular arthroscopic approach were followed up for a minimum of 6 months (average 23.7 months, range 6–48 months). The inclusion criteria included chronic ankle instability, without malalignment, low or moderate sports activity, failed conservative protocol, and without other pathology (fractures, subtalar instability, peroneal tendon dislocation). Patients with previous neuromuscular illnesses, active in professional sports, and with deformities were excluded. The group consisted of 39 male and 93 female patients, of average age 41.6 ± 15.1 years. Sports activity, represented as frequency

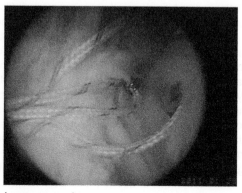

Fig. 8. Intra-articular knots are made.

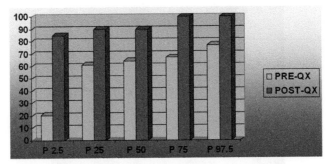

Fig. 9. AOFAS pre and post surgical intervention score.

of the event in a week, varied from none to 5 times a week, with an average of 1.96 per week. Duration of symptoms before the surgical procedure was, on average, 12.1. Including the associated abnormalities, anterolateral impingement was found in 117 patients (88.63%), synovitis in 29 (21.96%), osteochondral lesion type IIA (Ferkel classification) in 4 (3.03%), reflex dystrophy managed presurgically with pain control and rehabilitation in 1 (0.75%), and symptomatic hyperuricemia in 1 patient (0.75%). The preoperative AOFAS was 64 (range 25–77) and the postoperative AOFAS was 90 (range 85–100, $P<.01$).[21]

Complications found included scar tenderness, which was present in the first 3 patients (2.27%) at the level of the triple knot using nonabsorbable sutures, after which the technique was modified by using absorbable sutures. New inversion trauma was present in 6 patients (4.54%). In 4 patients this was managed conservatively with an ambulatory boot for 4 weeks followed by the rehabilitation protocol. Surgery was redone in 2 patients (1.51%), 1 with a medial malleoli avulsion type and 1 with lateral ligament damage, using bone anchors and the same technique.

Transient superficial peroneal nerve paresthesia was found in 1 patient (0.75%), which improved using pregabalin and capsaicin cream. No superficial or deep infection was found, nor was arthrofibrosis (**Fig. 9**).

SUMMARY

Chronic instability of the ankle and anterolateral impingement syndrome are abnormalities that present as a result of inversion and forced plantar-flexion traumas of the foot, despite strict conservative management in the ER and in rehabilitation. A conservative approach is always the first choice of treatment, including anti-inflammatory medications, rehabilitation and proprioception, infiltration with steroids in impingement cases, and use of orthotics, whose true effectiveness is the subject of multiple studies and much debate.[4,5] Good to excellent results can be obtained surgically with a minimally invasive approach, such as the arthroscopic technique presented herein. Such an approach is useful in managing a combination of conditions such as anterolateral impingement, synovitis, and osteochondral lesions of the talus. The method is easily reproducible, its learning curve is rapid, and it has the advantage of not preventing the use other arthroscopic methods, or open anatomic or nonanatomic methods (tendon transfers), in the case of failure. No nerve lesion was recorded, probably owing to the use of the security zone, and neither was there any arthrofibrosis, possibly related to the use of nonsteroidal anti-inflammatory medications in the immediate postsurgical period coupled with aggressive rehabilitation from the fourth week. The success of the technique is due to multidisciplinary team work leading to the ultimate achievement of patient satisfaction. This technique is not indicated for patients with a high sports demand or for sport professionals, until further biomechanical studies on its use and success are completed.

REFERENCES

1. Brooks SC, Potter BT, Raney JB. Treatment for partial tears of the lateral ligament of the ankle: a prospective trial. Br Med J 1981;282:606.
2. Ruth CJ. The surgical treatment of injuries of the fibular collateral ligaments of the ankle. J Bone Surg Am 1961;43:229.
3. McMasters PE. Treatment of ankle sprain: observations in more than five hundred cases. JAMA 1943;122:659.
4. Bosien RW, Staples OS, Rusell SW. Residual disability following acute ankle sprains. J Bone Joint Surg Am 1955;37:1237.
5. Freeman M. Instability of the foot after injuries of the lateral ligament of the ankle. J Bone Joint Surg Br 1965;47:669.
6. Bytin MJ, Fisher DA, Neuman L. Syndesmotic ankle sprains. Am J Sports Med 1991;19:294.
7. Conti SF, Stone DA. Chapter 8. Rehabilitation of fractures and sprains of the ankle. In: Sammarco GJ, editor. Rehabilitation of the foot and ankle. St Louis (MO): Mosby-Year Book, Inc; 1995:95–6.
8. Garrick JG. The frequency of injury, mechanism of injury and epidemiology of ankle sprains. Am J Sports Med 1977;5:241.
9. Gerstner JB. Lesiones de tobillo. In: en Echeverri A, Gerstner J, editors. Conceptos en traumatología. Cali (Colombia): Impresora Feriva S.A.; 1997:247–52.
10. Gould JS. Operative foot surgery. Philadelphia: Saunders; 1994.
11. Weber BJ. Lesiones traumáticas de la articulación del tobillo. Barcelona (Spain): Editorial Científico-Medica Barcelona; 1971.
12. Gerstner J, Gerstner JB. Manual de semiológia del aparato locomotor, 13ª Edición. Cali (Colombia): Impresora Feriva S.A.; 2011.
13. Myerson MS. Foot and ankle disorders. Philadelphia: W.B. Saunders Company; 2000.
14. Amendola A. Foot Fellow's review: controversies en diagnosis and management of syndesmosis injuries of the ankle. Foot Ankle 1992;13:92.
15. Becker H, Komischke A, Danz B, et al. Stress diagnostics of the sprained ankle: evaluation of the anterior drawer test with and without anaesthesia. Foot Ankle 1993;14:459.
16. Larsen E. Static or dynamic repair of chronic lateral ankle instability. Clin Orthop 1990;257:184.
17. Parisien JS. Techniques in therapeutic arthroscopy. New York: Raven Press; 1993.
18. Broström L. Sprained ankles, IV: surgical treatment of "chronic" ligament ruptures. Acta Chir Scand 1966;132:551–65.
19. Gould N. Repair of the lateral ligament of the ankle. Foot Ankle 1987;8:155.
20. Medveckyx M, Ong BC, Rokito AS, et al. Thermal capsular shrinkage: basic science and clinical applications. Arthroscopy 2001;17(6):624–35.
21. Siegol S. Estadística no parametrica. México (DF): Editorial Trivas; 1982.
22. Camu F. Valdecoxib, a COX-2-specific Inhibitor, is an efficacious opioid sparing analgesic in patients undergoing hip arthroplasty. Am J Ther 2002; 9:41–51.
23. Kitaoka H, Alexander I, Adelaar R, et al. Clinical rating systems for the ankle-hindfoot, midfoot, hallux and lesser toes. Foot Ankle Int 1994;15(7):349–53.

24. Corte-Real N, Moreira R. Arthroscopic repair of chronic lateral ankle instability. Foot Ankle Int 2009;30(3):213–7.
25. Nery C, Raduan F, Del Buono A, et al. Arthroscopic-assisted Broström-Gould for chronic ankle instability: a long-term follow-up. Am J Sports Med 2011;39(11): 2381–8.

Tendoscopy in Stage I Posterior Tibial Tendon Dysfunction

Gabriel Khazen, MD*, Cesar Khazen, MD

KEYWORDS

- Posterior tibial tendon • Dysfunction • Tendoscopy • Synovitis

KEY POINTS

- Stage I posterior tibial tendon dysfunction (PTTD) was defined by Johnson and Strom as tenosynovitis or tendinitis whereby tendon length remains normal, there is no hindfoot deformity, and diagnosis is basically clinical, characterized by swelling and tenderness posterior to the medial malleolus.
- Patients with stage I PTTD are first treated nonoperatively. If symptoms persist, surgical debridement and synovectomy has been suggested.
- Posterior tibial tendoscopic synovectomy is a minimally invasive and effective surgical procedure to treat patients with stage I PTTD. It has the advantages of less wound pain, and fewer scar and wound problems. If tendon tear is observed during tendoscopy, it must be repaired with nonabsorbable suture using a 3- or 4-cm incision.

Posterior tibial tendon dysfunction (PTTD)[1–6] is a wide-spectrum disease ranging from tenosynovitis to adult acquired flatfoot deformity. Stage I PTTD was defined by Johnson and Strom[3] as tenosynovitis or tendinitis whereby tendon length remains normal, there is no hindfoot deformity, and diagnosis is basically clinical, characterized by swelling and tenderness posterior to the medial malleolus caused by pitting edema[7] along the course of the posterior tibial tendon (PTT), which may radiate distally following the tendon. The PTT has a hypovascular zone[8] 40 mm proximal to the insertion of the tendon and 14 mm in length, and pain is often localized in this portion of the tendon.

In stage I PTTD,[3] tendon power might be normal and the patient can perform a single heel rise, sometimes with slight discomfort. This condition is often misdiagnosed as ankle sprain,[1] which delays correct diagnosis and early treatment that may improve symptoms, stop the disease process, and prevent the development of adult acquired flatfoot deformity.

The authors have nothing to disclose.
Unidad de Pié y Tobillo, Hospital de Clínicas Caracas, Caracas, Venezuela
* Corresponding author. Unidad de Pié y Tobillo, Hospital de Clínicas Caracas, Av Panteon, piso 4, cons 402, San Bernardino, Caracas, Venezuela.
E-mail address: gabrielkhazen@hotmail.com

Foot Ankle Clin N Am 17 (2012) 399–406
http://dx.doi.org/10.1016/j.fcl.2012.06.002
1083-7515/12/$ – see front matter © 2012 Elsevier Inc. All rights reserved.

Ultrasonography[9] and magnetic resonance imaging (MRI)[10] are valuable adjunctive diagnostic tools, and assist in achieving an accurate diagnosis of stage I PTTD. In a comparison of ultrasonography and MRI,[11] ultrasonography proved to be slightly less sensitive than MRI for PTT abnormality. The authors routinely order MRI for patients with suspected stage I PTTD.

Myerson and colleagues[12] determined 2 separate groups of patients with PTTD. The first group consists of younger patients with an average age of 30 years, with some form of systemic inflammatory disease (seronegative spondyloarthropathies). The second group comprises older patients with an average age of 55 years and long-standing microtrauma or overuse, which might be the source of dysfunction.

To analyze biomechanical and clinical factors[13] related to stage I PTTD, differences in arch height, ankle muscle strength, and biomechanical factors in individuals with stage I PTTD were investigated and compared with healthy individuals. The runners with PTTD demonstrated significantly lower seated arch height index and greater and prolonged peak rearfoot eversion angle during gait, compared with the healthy runners. The increased foot pronation is hypothesized to place greater strain on the posterior tibialis muscle, which may partially explain the progressive nature of this condition.

Patients with stage I PTTD are first treated nonoperatively with nonsteroidal anti-inflammatory drugs for 5 days, cryotherapy, local ultrasound, and a PTTD airlift brace (Aircast) for 3 to 6 months.[1,14–19] Alvarez and colleagues[19] suggested a protocol with an orthosis and high-repetition exercise program, aggressive plantarflexion activities, and gastrocsoleus tendon stretching. At 4 months, 83% of the 47 patients studied had successful subjective and functional outcomes. Kulig and colleagues[16] described a 10-week twice-daily, progressive eccentric tendon loading, calf-stretching program with orthoses, which was implemented by 10 early-stage tibialis posterior tendinopathy subjects. The subjects showed improvement in symptoms and function without changes in tendon morphology or neovascularization.

Patients with heel valgus and forefoot pronation that improve symptoms after conservative treatment may benefit from shoe modifications that tilt the hindfoot into slight varus.[20] Adding scaphoid support and a posteromedial sole wedge on a custom-made orthosis may take some tension off the PTT.

If symptoms persist, surgical debridement and synovectomy has been suggested.[1,4,17] Mann[21] recommended tenosynovectomy for early stage I PTTD lesions because synovitis can invade the tendon and cause degeneration and, possibly, tendon rupture. Myerson and colleagues[12] suggested considering tenosynovectomy after 3 months of conservative treatment in patients with tenosynovitis resulting from overuse or mechanical causes. Synovectomy should be considered earlier (after 6 weeks) in patients with seronegative disease.

Teasdall and Johnson[17] reported complete relief of symptoms or minor pain in 17 of 19 patients with stage I PTTD, after open debridement and synovectomy by a curvilinear incision along the medial ankle over the course of the posterior tibial tendon.[22–24] PTT debridement and synovectomy can be performed endoscopically. Chow and colleagues[23] suggested tendoscopic debridement for stage I PTTD to avoid wound problems such as wound infection, pain, scar contracture, and longer hospital stay, showing that it is a safe procedure capable of achieving effectiveness similar to that of the traditional open procedure, without complications.

The authors have performed PTT tendoscopic debridement for stage I PTTD in 9 patients since 2008, all but 1 of whom improved their symptoms and did not progress to stage II PTTD. Three patients had tendon tear and needed open repair.

POSTERIOR TIBIAL TENDON TENDOSCOPY
Surgical Technique

The authors routinely use the 2-portals technique as described by Van Dijk and colleagues[22,25]:

- The patient is placed in supine position; the procedure is always performed under ischemia.
- The operation can be performed under general or regional anesthesia.
- The PTT is examined and marked on the skin, using the medial malleolus and navicular as reference (**Fig. 1**).
- The 2 portals are placed over the tendon, the distal portal 2 cm proximal to the navicular insertion and the proximal portal 3 cm posterior and superior to the medial malleolus (**Fig. 2**).
- The incision is made through the skin and the tendon sheath is opened by blunt dissection with a hemostat.
- The 30° 2.7-mm arthroscope is introduced, and the tendon sheath is filled with saline (**Figs. 3** and **4**).
- The PTT is visualized from its insertion at the navicular up to 4 cm above the proximal portal, and inspected with the blunt probe. The tendon sheath is examined carefully.
- Synovectomy is performed with a small joint or 3.5-mm arthroscopic shaver system.
- At the end of the procedure, the portals are sutured.
- After tendoscopy, the patient is put on an airlift PTTD ankle brace (Aircast) for 6 weeks, for the first 2 weeks allowing partial weight bearing, then full weight bearing.
- Patients remain on a custom-made orthosis on their regular shoes, tilting the hindfoot into slight varus, with a scaphoid support and posteromedial sole wedge, to protect the tendon.

Posterior Tibial Tendon Tear

If there is any important PTT tear visualized during tendoscopy (**Fig. 5**):

- Tendon sheath must be opened via a 3- or 4-cm incision and the tear repaired.
- Diseased tendon should be removed and fissures debrided, and the gap repaired with 2-0 nonabsorbable sutures (Ethibond).

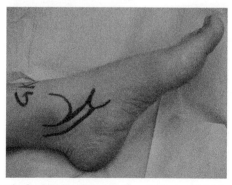

Fig. 1. Surgical landmarks for PTT tendoscopy. The posterior tibial tendon is marked in the skin, using medial malleolus and navicular as reference.

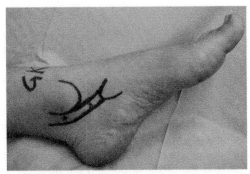

Fig. 2. Surgical landmarks for PTT tendoscopy. The 2 portals are placed over the tendon, the distal portal 2 cm proximal to the navicular insertion and the proximal portal 3 cm posterior and superior to the medial malleolus.

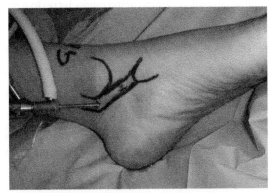

Fig. 3. The 30° 2.7-mm arthroscope is introduced. The posterior tibial tendon is visualized by the 2 portals, first via the navicular insertion.

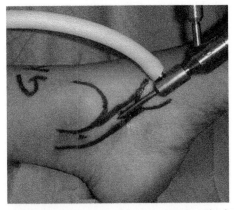

Fig. 4. The 30° 2.7-mm arthroscope is introduced. The posterior tibial tendon is visualized up to 4 cm above the proximal portal.

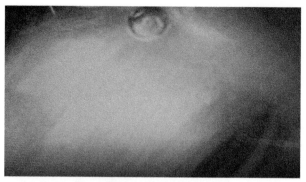

Fig. 5. PTT tear visualized during tendoscopy.

- The tendon sheath is left open to avoid scarring (**Figs. 6** and **7**).
- After tendon repair, the patient is put on a non–weight-bearing walking boot for 3 weeks, and partial weight bearing is allowed for 3 weeks.
- At 6 weeks after surgery, an airlift PTTD ankle brace (Aircast) is indicated for 6 weeks.

The authors added subtalar arthrosis for this patient to protect and take some tension off the repaired tendon, but the implant had to be removed at 6 months after surgery in 2 of the 3 patients because of pain and discomfort in the sinus tarsi.

RESULTS

Chow and colleagues[23] reported no complications after tendoscopy in stage I PTTD. All their patients were completely pain free and had normal strength of tendon action,

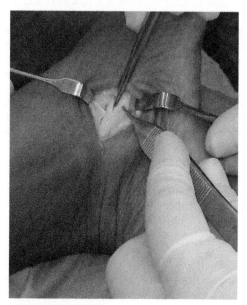

Fig. 6. Tendon repair. The tendon sheath most be open via a 3- or 4-cm incision and the tear repaired. Diseased tendon should be removed and fissures debrided.

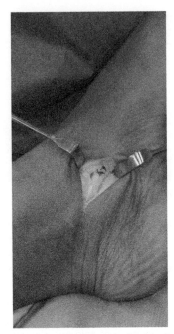

Fig. 7. Tendon repair. The gap is repaired with 2-0 nonabsorbable sutures.

as demonstrated by single heel rise test at 2 months after surgery. The advantages of this procedure are a cosmetically very well-accepted scar (only 2 4-mm scars), less wound pain, and fewer complications than with the open procedure. None of their patients progressed to disease stage II or above when followed up for 4 to 30 months (average 17 months). Patients resumed work at a 10 weeks and resumed sports after 6 months.

The authors have performed tendoscopic debridement for stage I PTTD in 9 patients since 2008, all but 1 of whom showed subjective and objective improvement of their symptoms and did not progress to stage II PTTD within 3 years (10–38 months of follow up). The one unsatisfied patient did not have a tendon tear. This patient progressed to stage II PTTD and needed hindfoot reconstruction. Three patients had tendon tears and needed open repair; only 1 of these 3 patients manifested discomfort and skin issues after surgery, which settled down at 8 weeks postoperatively. Tendoscopic synovectomy patients resumed work at between 4 and 6 weeks, and patients with tendon tear returned to work at 10 weeks.

Funk and colleagues[6] reviewed 9 patients undergoing tenosynovectomy with and without repair of a longitudinal split tear of the tendon. All patients showed subjective and objective improvement. Pain was rated as absent or minor in 8 of 9 (89%) patients, with 8 patients having the capability to perform a single heel rise postoperatively.

SUMMARY

Stage I PTTD was defined by Johnson and Strom as tenosynovitis or tendinitis whereby tendon length remains normal, there is no hindfoot deformity, and diagnosis is basically clinical, characterized by swelling and tenderness posterior to the medial malleolus. The PTT has a hypovascular zone 40 mm proximal to the insertion of the tendon and 14 mm in length. Pain often is localized to this portion of the tendon.

Tendon power might be normal, and the patient can perform single heel rise, sometimes with slight discomfort.

This condition is often misdiagnosed as ankle sprain, which delays correct diagnosis and early treatment that may improve symptoms, stop the disease process, and prevent the development of adult acquired flatfoot deformity. Ultrasonography is a valuable adjunctive diagnostic tool for stage I PTTD, but the authors always indicate MRI for accurate diagnosis in such patients.

Patients with stage I PTTD are first treated nonoperatively with nonsteroidal anti-inflammatory drugs for 5 days, cryotherapy, local ultrasound, and a PTTD airlift brace (Aircast) for 3 to 6 months. If symptoms persist, surgical debridement and synovectomy has been suggested.

PTT tendoscopic synovectomy is a minimally invasive and effective surgical procedure to treat patients with stage I PTTD. It has the advantages of less wound pain, and fewer scar and wound problems. If tendon tear is observed during tendoscopy, it must be repaired with nonabsorbable sutures using a 3- or 4-cm incision.

REFERENCES

1. Bare AA, Haddad SL. Tenosynovitis of the posterior tibial tendon. Foot Ankle Clin 2001;6:37–66.
2. Johnson KA. Tibialis posterior tendon rupture. Clin Orthop 1983;177:140–7.
3. Johnson KA, Strom DE. Tibialis posterior tendon dysfunction. Clin Orthop 1989; 239:197–206.
4. Beals TC, Pomeroy GC, Manoli A 2nd. Posterior tendon insufficiency: diagnosis and treatment. J Am Acad Orthop Surg 1999;7(2):112–8.
5. Trnka HJ. Dysfunction of the tendon of tibialis posterior. J Bone Joint Surg Br 2004;7:939–46.
6. Funk DA, Cass JR, Johnson KA. Acquired adult flat foot secondary to posterior tibial-tendon pathology. J Bone Joint Surg Am 1986;68:95–101.
7. DeOrio JK, Shapiro SA, McNeil RB, et al. Validity of the posterior tibial edema sign in posterior tibial tendon dysfunction. Foot Ankle Int 2011;32(2):189–92.
8. Holmes GB, Mann RA. Possible epidemiological factors associated with rupture of the posterior tibial tendon. Foot Ankle Int 1992;13:70–9.
9. Miller SD, van Holsbeeck M, Boruta PM. Ultrasound in the diagnosis of the diagnosis of the posterior tibial tendon pathology. Foot Ankle Int 1996;17(9): 555–8.
10. Chen YJ, Liang SC. Diagnostic efficacy of ultrasonography in stage I posterior tibial tendon dysfunction: sonographic-surgical correlation. J Ultrasound Med 1997;16(6):417–23.
11. Nallamshetty L, Nazarian LN, Schweitzer ME, et al. Evaluation of posterior tibial pathology: comparison of sonography and MR imaging. Skeletal Radiol 2005; 34(7):375–80.
12. Myerson M, Solomon G, Shereff M. Posterior tibial tendon dysfunction: its association with seronegative inflammatory disease. Foot Ankle 1989;9:219–25.
13. Rabbito M, Pohl MB, Humble N, et al. Biomechanical and clinical factors related to stage I posterior tibial tendon dysfunction. J Orthop Sports Phys Ther 2011; 41(10):776–84.
14. Sferra JJ, Rosenberg GA. Nonoperative treatment of posterior tibial tendon pathology. Foot Ankle Clin 1997;2:261–73.
15. Augustin JF, Lin SS, Berberian WS, et al. Non-operative treatment of adult acquired flatfoot with the Arizona brace. Foot Ankle Clin 2003;8(3):491–502.

16. Kulig K, Lederhaus ES, Reischl S, et al. Effect of eccentric exercise program for early tibialis posterior tendinopathy. Foot Ankle Int 2009;30(9):877–85.
17. Teasdall RD, Johnson KA. Surgical treatment of stage I posterior tibial tendon dysfunction. Foot Ankle Int 1994;15(12):646–8.
18. Crates JM, Richardson EG. Treatment of stage I posterior tibial tendon dysfunction with medial soft tissue procedures. Clin Orthop Relat Res 1999;(365):46–9.
19. Alvarez RG, Marini A, Schmitt C, et al. Stage I and II posterior tibial tendon dysfunction treated by a structured nonoperative management protocol: an orthosis and exercise program. Foot Ankle Int 2006;27(1):2–8.
20. Kaye RA, Jahss MH. Tibialis posterior: a review of anatomy and biomechanics in relation to support of the medial longitudinal arch. Foot Ankle 1991;11:244–7.
21. Mann RA. Acquired flatfoot in adults. Clin Orthop 1983;181:46–51.
22. Bulstra GH, Olsthoorn P, Van Dijk CN. Tendoscopy of the posterior tibial tendon. Foot Ankle Clin 2006;11:421–7.
23. Chow HT, Kwok BC, Tun HL. Tendoscopic debridement for stage I posterior tibial tendon dysfunction. Knee Surg Sports Traumatol Arthrosc 2005;13:695–8.
24. Wertheimer SJ, Weber CA, Loder BG. The role of endoscopy in treatment of posterior tibial synovitis. J Foot Ankle Surg 1995;34(1):15–22.
25. Van Dijk CN, Kort N, Scholten PE. Tendoscopy of the posterior tibial tendon. Arthroscopy 1997;13(6):692–8.

Subtle Lisfranc Joint Ligament Lesions: Surgical Neoligamentplasty Technique

Caio Nery, MD*, Cibele Réssio, MD, José Felipe Marion Alloza, MD

KEYWORDS

- Lisfranc injury • Lisfranc ligament • Tarsometatarsal lesion

KEY POINTS

- The treatment of intercuneiform and tarsometatarsal joint fracture dislocations is still controversial and, despite appropriate treatments, a considerable number of patients develop painful osteoarthritis.
- This article presents a new surgical technique to reconstruct the ligamentous complex of the region based on the reproduction of its anatomy and isometrics.
- By making strategic bone tunnels in the cuneiforms and metatarsal bases, the harvesting of the extensor digitorum longus tendon reinforced by an unabsorbable suture gives rise to a neoligament that keeps the joints mobile and flexible.
- The neoligamentplasty is a valid alternative to the classic treatment of subtle intercuneiform and tarsometatarsal joint lesions.

INTRODUCTION

Isolated tarsometatarsal ligament lesions are caused by indirect low-energy forces combined with rotational movements applied to the foot.[1] Although this is a rare condition, it can lead to poor functional results with the rapid development of arthritis of the joints involved.[2–19]

Some investigators state that a great number of these lesions are misdiagnosed or overlooked and consider them worrisome.[10]

The treatment options found in the literature include closed reduction with a non–weight-bearing cast,[2,12,17] closed reduction with percutaneous K-wire fixation,[1,4,6,9,11,17,20] open reduction with internal fixation with screws,[2,3,8,10] bridge plates,[21] suture-button fixation, and arthrodesis.[20,22–32]

The gold-standard method in the literature to deal with these lesions is open reduction and internal fixation with screws, but, in recent publications, the good results of this method are questioned and midterm follow-up has detected painful arthritis in a significant percentage of patients.[32]

The authors have nothing to disclose.
Federal University of São Paulo-UNIFESP, Escola Paulista de Medicina, São Paulo, Brazil
* Corresponding author. Avenida Rouxinol 404, 2nd Floor 04516-000, São Paulo, SP, Brazil.
E-mail addresses: caionery@uol.com.br; caionerymd@gmail.com

Even in joints with restricted movements, such as those in the tarsal and tarsome-tatarsal regions, it is therefore advisable to maintain functional mobility and stability. We proposed a technique based on anatomic reduction, including the resection of any remaining ligament, and anatomic reconstruction principles of the intercuneiform and tarsometatarsal ligaments.[23–26]

CLINICAL FINDINGS

The typical patient complains of pain in the midfoot after a foot sprain when running or playing on a yielding surface or after twisting the forefoot while stepping in a hole on the ground. In acute cases, dorsal midfoot swelling and ecchymosis are found in the plantar aspect of the foot (**Fig. 1**).The ankle is usually stable and pain free with no swelling or ecchymosis. It is important to perform a thorough clinical examination to avoid mistaking a foot sprain for an ankle sprain, a common (65%) and dangerous mistake.[25]

According to Jeffreys,[1] the pure tarsometatarsal ligament lesion injury pattern depends on the application of rotational forces to a plantar-flexed foot while the fore-foot is firmly fixed on the ground. It is important to clarify the direction of the forces applied to the foot during the trauma, which shows which structures are involved: when inversion forces are applied, the dorsal and interosseous ligaments may be torn; when eversion forces act, the plantar and interosseous ligaments may be affected. The application of rotational maneuvers to the forefoot while the hindfoot is kept stable is a useful tool to clarify traumatic movements (**Fig. 2**).

In a couple of weeks, the pain and swelling subside, but the patient is still unable to walk long distances or stand on tiptoe.[20,25,28] Wearing shoes, especially high-heeled shoes, is uncomfortable or even impossible.

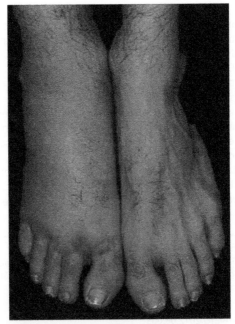

Fig. 1. A patient 2 days after a sprain in the right foot.

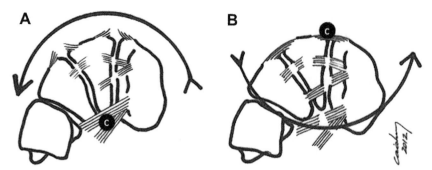

Fig. 2. Injury pattern. (*A*) Inversion force with external rotation of the midfoot. The center of rotation (c) coincides with the ligaments of the plantar layer, which are preserved. The dorsal layer ligaments suffer first, followed by the ligaments of the interosseous layer. (*B*) Eversion force with internal rotation of the midfoot. The center of rotation (c) coincides with the ligaments of the dorsal layer, which are preserved. The plantar layer ligaments suffer first, followed by the ligaments of the interosseous layer.

PLAIN RADIOGRAPHS

As a general rule, it is important to obtain anteroposterior and lateral standing weight-bearing views of both feet to identify any articular incongruence or tarsal bone fractures.

The candle-flame sign, described by Turco,[16] is a diastasis (>5 mm) between the medial and intermediate cuneiforms, between the medial cuneiform and the second metatarsal base, or between the bases of the first and second metatarsals, which represents an important ligament lesion. However, only 55% of patients with an important tarsometatarsal lesion showed radiographic signals in plain standing radiographs.[25] For a complete radiographic analysis of a patient, oblique radiographs are recommended to check the congruency of the tarsometatarsal joints (**Fig. 3**).

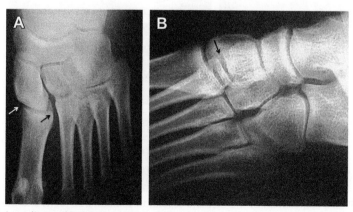

Fig. 3. Plain radiographs. (*A*) The candle-flame sign that is a diastasis between the first and second cuneiform bones (*black arrow*). Subluxation of the first tarsometatarsal joint is also visible (*white arrow*). (*B*) In the oblique view, joint congruency can be checked. In this example, there is a subluxation of the second tarsometatarsal joint (*arrow*).

A classification system proposed by Nunley and Verullo's[25] addresses subtle soft tissue injuries that affect the ligament structures with or without small fleck or avulsed fractures. According to these investigators:

- Stage I consists of a tarsometatarsal ligament sprain without diastasis between the bones or loss of the medial arch height on weight-bearing radiographs; the Lisfranc complex is stable.
- Stage II shows diastasis of up to 5 mm between the medial cuneiform and the base of the second metatarsal, but there is no loss of the medial arch height; the Lisfranc ligament may be torn, but there still are enough ligaments to keep the Lisfranc complex in the correct place.
- Stage III results in diastasis greater than 5 mm and reduction of the medial arch height; both the Lisfranc and the Y plantar ligament are injured.

MAGNETIC RESONANCE IMAGING

Magnetic resonance imaging (MRI) is the best method to identify torn ligaments, joint displacements, and possible avulsion fractures. In our experience, MRI has high sensitivity and specificity in the detection of ligament injuries of the tarsometatarsal region and is helpful in those patients with a history of foot sprain, regardless of how long ago the injury occurred (**Fig. 4**).

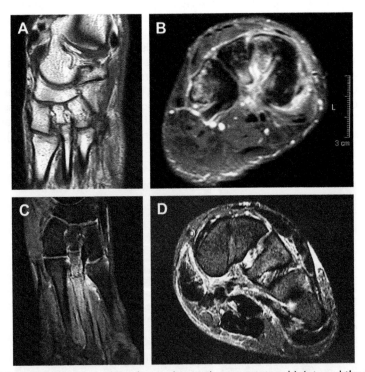

Fig. 4. MRI. (*A*) Subluxation of the first and second tarsometatarsal joints and the torn Lisfranc ligament. (*B*) Coronal image showing the deep hypersignal indicating the involvement of the ligaments of the plantar layer. (*C*) The Lisfranc ligament was avulsed from the metaphysis of the second metatarsal. There is a fracture at the base of the same metatarsal. (*D*) This coronal image shows an important diastasis between C2 and C3 after a sprained foot.

To take advantage of the quality of MRI, an understanding of the tarsal and tarso-metatarsal anatomy is of the utmost importance. Both the morphology of the bones (cuneiforms, metatarsals, and cuboid bases) and the dense ligamentous attachments play an important role in the physiology of these joints and may influence the decision-making process, as well as the surgical planning.

ANATOMY

The 3 cuneiform bones, as well as the bases of the first, second, and third metatarsals, are wedge-shaped and, together with the fourth and fifth proximal metaphysis and the cuboid bone, form a balanced arch in the frontal plane of the midfoot. The keystone of this stable arrangement seems to be the base of the second metatarsal, but the liga-ment complex of the region is important, because the rationale of the surgical treat-ment is based on it.

There are 3 ligament layers connecting the cuneiforms and the cuboid to the meta-tarsal bases: the dorsal, interosseous, and plantar ligaments.[33]

Dorsal Layer

Two dorsal, rectangular, transversally oriented ligament-tissue bands connect the first to the second and the second to the third cuneiforms at the medial portion of the tarsal region (**Fig. 5**). A broad, triangular, fragile tissue band occupies the space between the lateral cuneiform and the cuboid.

There are several dorsal tarsometatarsal ligaments, but some of them are just a thickening of the articular capsule. The base of the first metatarsal is connected to the first cuneiform by a strong dorsomedial ligament (see **Fig. 4**A, D). The base of the second metatarsal is connected to the dorsum of the medial (first), middle (second), and lateral (third) cuneiforms by 3 ligaments. The base of the third metatarsal is connected to the dorsum of the lateral cuneiform by a dorsal ligament, and the bases of the fourth and fifth metatarsal bones are connected to the cuboid by dorso-lateral ligaments.

Interosseous Layer

Two interosseous ligaments connect the 3 cuneiform bones. Both are short and strong transversely oriented bands uniting the cuneiforms. The medial interosseous ligament is located on the posterior half of the lateral surface, at least 8 mm posterior to the anterior border of the bone (see **Fig. 4**B). The lateral interosseous cuneiform ligament is located anterior to the intercuneiform articular surfaces.

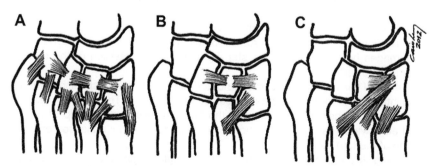

Fig. 5. Ligaments of the intercuneiform and tarsometatarsal joints. (*A*) Dorsal layer; (*B*) in-terosseous layer; (*C*) plantar layer.

The most important and strongest interosseous tarsometatarsal ligament is the Lisfranc ligament between the medial cuneiform and the base of the second metatarsal. The Lisfranc ligament arises from the lateral surface of the first cuneiform, just under the articular surface of the intermediate cuneiform and distal to the intercuneiform ligament. It runs obliquely outward and downward and inserts in the lower half of the medial surface of the second metatarsal base, about 5 mm from the proximal end of the bone.

Plantar Layer

On the plantar surface, there is a short and strong ligament that originates on the posterolateral corner of the medial cuneiform and inserts in the crest of the second cuneiform: the plantar intercuneiform ligament (see **Fig. 4**C).

The medial cuneiform is attached to the base of the first metatarsal by a broad ligament that originates from the plantar aspect of the cuneiform and inserts in the lateral half of the first metatarsal base.

The strongest plantar ligament, considered the keystone of the tarsometatarsal arch,[1,4] originates from the lateral surface of the medial cuneiform and consists of 2 bands: the superficial band is strong and thick and inserts strongly in the base of the third metatarsal; the deep band is weaker and inserts in the base of second metatarsal (Y ligament).

There are no plantar ligaments between the second cuneiform and the second metatarsal.

The stronger ligament is the Lisfranc ligament (C1–M2) in the interosseous layer, followed by the Y plantar ligament (C1–M2+M3), and then by the more delicate dorsal layer. The lateral Lisfranc joint (fourth and fifth), provided with weaker and thinner ligaments, is less prone to ligament injuries because of its mobility and flexibility.[34]

SURGICAL TECHNIQUE

The region of the intercuneiforms and tarsometatarsal joints is exposed through a transverse dorsal incision. To reduce the risk of injuries, the dorsal pedis artery and the deep peroneal nerve are identified and retracted.[35–38] Alternatively, 2 or 3 longitudinal skin incisions can be used, but their location must be precise to allow for the correct positioning of the bone tunnels. It is important for the outcome of the surgery to identify all torn structures. To help in the recognition of the ruptured tissues, rotational force can be applied to the forefoot to reproduce the traumatic mechanism.

Removing all ligament remains is one of the most important tasks in this technique, especially in the interosseous layer,[25–30] because this favors the anatomic reduction of the joints and prevents the persistent pain observed in abandoned patients or those treated by closed reduction and percutaneous screw fixation (**Fig. 6**). Magnetic resonance images help in planning the step-by-step surgical revision of the anatomic structures involved.

The result of this meticulous revision and debridement is the reestablishment of the normal intercuneiform and tarsometatarsal joint relationship. The next step is to find the correct tridimensional orientation of the bone tunnels with the help of a C-arm and a free K-wire. Then, 3 mm drill holes are made to reproduce the isometrics and anatomy of the torn ligaments.

According to the anatomic orientation of the original ligaments, there are 3 main tunnels that have to be made before reconstructing the regional ligament anatomy (**Fig. 7**).[25]

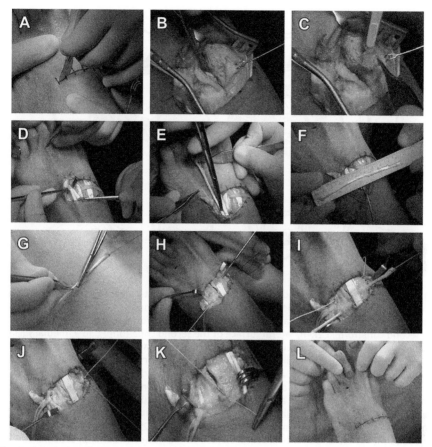

Fig. 6. Surgical technique. (*A*) Dorsal transverse incision. (*B*) Inventory of the lesions. (*C*) Removal of torn ligaments. (*D*) Isolation of the third EDL tendon. (*E*) Proximal dissection of the third EDL tendon. (*F*) Harvesting the tendon. (*G*) Adding sutures to reinforce the tendon. (*H*) Drilling the bone tunnels. (*I*) The neoligament driven through the tunnels. (*J*) Tensioning the suture and the harvested tendon. (*K*) Closing all incision layers. (*L*) Final aspect of the foot after the skin closure.

First Transverse Tunnel

The first transverse tunnel runs from the deep point of the first cuneiform medial surface depression to the midpoint of the third cuneiform dorsolateral border. When correctly oriented, this tunnel crosses the geometric center of the first cuneiform, the distal half of the second cuneiform, and the geometric center of the third cuneiform, preserving all articular surfaces of the 3 bones. This tunnel is intended to recreate the cuneiform interosseous ligaments.

Second Oblique Tunnel

The second oblique tunnel runs from the medial surface of the first cuneiform to the proximal metaphysis of the second metatarsal and is intended to reproduce the Lisfranc ligament. When correctly oriented, this tunnel crosses the contact region between the first cuneiform and the base of the second metatarsal.

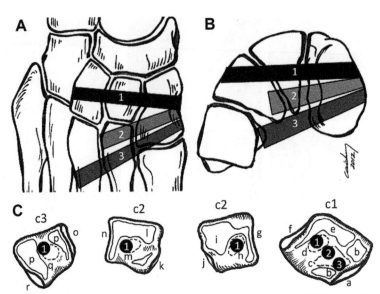

Fig. 7. Anatomic landmarks and positioning of the 3 bone tunnels. (*A*) Orientation of the tunnels in the transversal plane. (*B*) Orientation of the tunnels in the coronal plane. (*C*) Cuneiform bones: C1a–f, lateral surface of the first cuneiform; C2g–j, medial surface of the second cuneiform; C2k–n, lateral surface of the second cuneiform; C3o–r, medial surface of the third cuneiform. a, Articular surface for the first metatarsal; b, articular surface for the second metatarsal; c, insertional zone of the Lisfranc ligament; d, insertional zone of inter-cuneiform C1 to C2 ligament; e, articular surface to the second cuneiform; f, articular surface to the navicular bone; g, articular surface to the navicular bone; h, insertional zone of inter-cuneiform C1 to C2 ligament; i, articular surface to the first cuneiform; j, articular surface to the second metatarsal; k, articular surface to the second metatarsal; l, articular surface to the third cuneiform; m, insertional zone of intercuneiform C2 to C3 ligament; n, articular surface to the navicular bone; o, articular surface to the navicular bone; p, articular surface to the second cuneiform; q, insertional zone of intercuneiform C2 to C3 ligament; r, articular surface to the third metatarsal; 1, drill hole for the first tunnel; 2, drill hole for the second tunnel; 3, drill hole for the third tunnel.

Third Plantar Tunnel

The third plantar tunnel is also the most anterior tunnel, and runs obliquely from the first cuneiform to the base of the third metatarsal, reproducing the deep plantar ligaments (see **Fig. 7**).

It is not usually necessary to rely on the 3 tunnels described. To achieve the best and most stable correction possible, the surgeon must decide which tunnels will be needed and the best sequence to drive the harvested tendon into the tunnels. Preoperative planning is important, based on the clinical, radiological, and MRI findings. It is sometimes necessary to have short accessory tunnels connecting the main tunnels to stabilize the first cuneometatarsal joint or reinforce superficial layer ligaments.

To do this neoligamentplasty, we recommend harvesting the third extensor digitorum longus (EDL), reinforced by a 2.0 fiber-wire suture. Care must be taken in the harvesting of the EDL because it is necessary to have at least 9 cm of tendon tissue to complete the procedure as described.

The neoligament is driven trough the tunnels with the help of a tendon passer, and the correct tension is applied at the ends of the sutures to ensure the stability and flexibility of the joints. Before considering the completion of the procedure, the supination-pronation maneuver is repeated to check the efficiency and accuracy of the construct. We always try to hide the knots between the bones, in the interosseous musculature, or inside the tunnels.

The incision is closed in the usual manner and a short neutral leg splint is used for 3 weeks. The skin sutures are removed on the 21st postoperative day. The patient is submitted to an 8-week non–weight-bearing period followed by 3 months of rehabilitation.

SUMMARY

The results achieved with this technique after a mean follow-up of 8 years (85% excellent and good results[25]) allow neoligamentplasty to be considered as a viable alternative to the classic procedures in the treatment of subtle intercuneiform and tarsometatarsal joint lesions.

REFERENCES

1. Aitken AP, Poulson D. Dislocations of the tarsometatarsal joint. J Bone Joint Surg Am 1963;45(2):246–60.
2. Collett HS, Hood TK, Andrews RE. Tarsometatarsal fracture dislocations. Surg Gynecol Obstet 1958;106:623–6.
3. Faciszewski T, Burks RT, Manaster BJ. Subtle injuries of the Lisfranc joint. J Bone Joint Surg Am 1990;72(10):1519–22.
4. Goossens M, Stoop N. Lisfranc's fracture-dislocations: etiology, radiology and results of treatment. A review of 20 cases. Clin Orthop Relat Res 1983;176:154–62.
5. Groshar D, Alperson M, Mendes DG, et al. Bone scintigraphy findings in Lisfranc joint injury. Foot Ankle 1995;16(11):710–1.
6. Hardcastle PH, Reschauer R, Kutscha-Lissberg E, et al. Injuries to the tarsometatarsal joint. J Bone Joint Surg Br 1982;64(3):349–56.
7. Jeffreys TE. Lisfranc's fracture-dislocation. J Bone Joint Surg Br 1963;45(3):546–51.
8. Lynch JR, Cooperstein LA, DiGioia AM. Plantar medial subluxation of the medial cuneiform: case report of an uncommon variant of the Lisfranc injury. Foot Ankle 1995;16(5):299–301.
9. Markowitz HD, Chase M, Whitelaw GP. Isolated injury of the second tarsometatarsal joint. Clin Orthop Relat Res 1989;248:210–2.
10. Myerson MS, Fisher RT, Burgess AR, et al. Fracture dislocations of the tarsometatarsal joints: end results correlated with pathology and treatment. Foot Ankle 1986;6(5):225–42.
11. Morris KL, Giacopelli JA, Granoff DP. Medial column instability in the Lisfranc's fracture dislocation injury. J Foot Surg 1991;30(5):513–23.
12. Narat JK. An unusual case of dislocation of metatarsal bones. Am J Surg 1929;6(2):239–41.
13. Pelland PO. Complete dislocation of the bases metatarsals, without fracture. J Bone Joint Surg 1935;17:214–6.
14. Quénu E, Küss G. Étude sur les luxations du métatarse (luxations métatarso-tarsiennes). Rev Chir 1909;39:281–336, 720–91, 1093–134. [in French].
15. Shapiro MS, Wascher DC, Finerman GA. Rupture of Lisfranc's ligament in athletes. Am J Sports Med 1994;22(5):687–91.
16. Turco VJ. Diastasis of first and second tarsometatarsal rays: a cause of pain in the foot. Bull N Y Acad Med 1973;49:222–5.

17. Vuori JP, Aro HT. Lisfranc joint injuries: trauma mechanisms and associated injuries. J Trauma 1993;35(1):40–5.
18. Wilson DW. Injuries of the tarso-metatarsal joints. J Bone Joint Surg Br 1972; 54(4):677–86.
19. Yamashita F, Sakakida K, Hara K, et al. Diastasis between the medial and the intermediate cuneiforms. J Bone Joint Surg Br 1993;75(1):156–7.
20. Nery C, Barroco R, Magalhães AA, et al. Diástase traumática dos ossos cuneiformes do tarso. Revista Brasileira de Ortopedia 1996;31(7):531–6 [in Galician].
21. Nery C, Réssio C, Alloza JF. Lesões sutís das articulações intercuneiformes e tarsometatärsicas tratadas através da neoligamentoplastia. Revista da Associação Brasileira de Tornozelo e Pé 2007;1(1):51–8 [in Portuguese].
22. Nery C, Réssio C, Alloza JF. Neoligamentplasty for the treatment of subtle ligament lesions of the intercuneiform and tarsometatarsal joints. Tech Foot Ankle Surg 2010;9(3):92–9.
23. Nery C, Réssio C, Alloza JF. Técnica quirúrgica: neoligamentoplastia para el tratamiento de las lesions ligamentarias de las articulaciones intercineanas y tarsometatarsianas. Revista de la Federación Latinoamericana de Medicina y Cirugia de La Pierna y Pie 2011;2(3):108–12 [in Spanish].
24. DeOrio M, Erickson M, Usuelli FG, et al. Lisfranc injuries in sport. Foot Ankle Clin 2009;14:169–86.
25. Nunley JA, Vertullo CJ. Classification, investigation, and management of midfoot sprains: Lisfranc injuries in the athlete. Am J Sports Med 2002;30:871–8.
26. Granberry WM, Lipscomb PR. Dislocation of the tarsometatarsal joints. Surg Gynecol Obstet 1962;114:467–9.
27. Aranow MS. Treatment of the missed Lisfranc injury. Foot Ankle Clin 2006;11(1): 127–42.
28. Panchbhavi VK, Vallurupalli S, Yang J, et al. Screw fixation compared with suture-button fixation of isolated Lisfranc ligament injuries. J Bone Joint Surg Am 2009; 91(5):1143–8.
29. Coetzee JC. Making sense of Lisfranc injuries. Foot Ankle Clin 2008;13(4):695–704.
30. Desmond EA, Chou LB. Current concepts review: Lisfranc injuries. Foot Ankle Int 2006;27(8):653–60.
31. Henning JA, Jones CB, Sietsema DL, et al. Open reduction internal fixation versus primary arthrodesis for Lisfranc injuries: a prospective randomized study. Foot Ankle Int 2009;30(10):913–22.
32. Sarrafian SK. Anatomy of the foot and ankle. Descriptive, topographic, functional. 2nd edition. Pennsylvania: Lippincott Co.; 1993. p. 203–10.
33. Johnson A, Hill K, Ward J, et al. Anatomy of the Lisfranc ligament. Foot Ankle Spec 2008;1(1):19–23.
34. Wiley JJ. The mechanism of tarso-metatarsal joint injuries. J Bone Joint Surg Br 1971;53(3):474–82.
35. Kaar S, Femino J, Morag Y. Lisfranc joint displacement following sequential ligament sectioning. J Bone Joint Surg Am 2007;89(10):2225–32.
36. Raikin SM, Elias I, Dheer S, et al. Prediction of midfoot instability in the subtle Lisfranc injury. Comparison of magnetic resonance imaging with intraoperative findings. J Bone Joint Surg Am 2009;91(4):892–9.
37. MacMahon PJ, Dheer S, Raikin SM, et al. MRI of injuries to the first interosseous cuneometatarsal (Lisfranc) ligament. Skeletal Radiol 2009;38(3):255–60.
38. Mann RA, Prieskorn D, Sobel M. Mid-tarsal and TMT arthrodesis for primary degenerative osteoarthrosis or osteoarthrosis after trauma. J Bone Joint Surg Am 1996;78:1376–82.

Pull-Out Technique for Plantar Plate Repair of the Metatarsophalangeal Joint

José A.V. Sanhudo, MD[a],*, João L. Ellera Gomes, MD, PhD[b]

KEYWORDS

- Crossover toe • Plantar plate • Second metatarsophalangeal joint • Instability

KEY POINTS

- The plantar plate provides cushion to the metatarsal head, and is the most important structure for stability of the metatarsophalangeal joint (MTPJ).
- Plantar plate rupture is a common cause of forefoot pain, multiplanar malalignment, subluxation, or dislocation of the MTPJ.
- A group of factors seems to be associated to the development of the lesion known as crossover, which features sagittal and horizontal plane instability.
- Inflammatory arthritis, such as rheumatoid arthritis, or trauma, may also precipitate MTPJ destabilization of the lesser toes.

INTRODUCTION

The plantar plate provides cushion to the metatarsal head, and is the most important structure for stability of the metatarsophalangeal joint (MTPJ). Plantar plate rupture is a common cause of forefoot pain, multiplanar malalignment, subluxation, or disloca-tion of the MTPJ. A group of factors such as sagittal and horizontal plane instability, seems to be associated to the development of the lesion. The lesion is most commonly seen at the second ray, especially in the presence of index minus, and is often associated with hallux valgus or hallux rigidus.[1] Inflammatory arthritis, such as rheumatoid arthritis, or trauma, may also precipitate metatarsophalangeal joint desta-bilization of the lesser toes.

ANATOMY AND BIOMECHANICS

At the dorsal aspect of the MTPJ, the extensor digitorum longus (EDL) tendon is cen-trally located, splitting into 3 portions over the proximal phalanx: the central portion

[a] Department of Orthopaedic Surgery, Mãe de Deus Hospital, Rua José de Alencar 286, Porto Alegre, RS, 90880-480, Brazil; [b] Department of Orthopaedic and Traumatology, HCPA, Universidade Federal do Rio Grande do Sul, Rua Ramiro Barcelos 2350, Porto Alegre, RS, 90035-000, Brazil
* Corresponding author.
E-mail address: jsanhudo@ceotrs.com.br

Foot Ankle Clin N Am 17 (2012) 417–424
http://dx.doi.org/10.1016/j.fcl.2012.06.004
1083-7515/12/$ – see front matter © 2012 Elsevier Inc. All rights reserved.

attaches to the base of the middle phalanx, and the 2 adjacent portions blend over the dorsal aspect of that phalanx and attach to the base of the distal phalanx. A fibroaponeurotic apparatus extends from the MTPJ plantar region and proximal phalanx base to the dorsal region, surrounding and centrally stabilizing the EDL. The EDL does not have any proximal phalanx attachment, but acts through that fibroaponeurotic apparatus. The proximal phalanx is literally suspended (dorsiflexed) by the action of EDL over it. Besides MTPJ dorsiflexion, the EDL tendon may cause extension of the proximal (PIPJ) and distal (DIPJ) interphalangeal joints, as long as the proximal phalanx is in either neutral or plantar flexion position. Dorsiflexion of the proximal phalanx assures that EDL excursion is insufficient to exert tension onto the middle and distal phalanges. This concept is important in understanding the detrimental effect of high heels, which keep the proximal phalanx dorsiflexed, thus reducing or even nullifying the action of EDL onto the interphalangeal joints.[2–5]

Underneath, the MTPJ is stabilized by the joint capsule and the plantar aponeurosis, together forming the plantar plate. This structure is made of longitudinally oriented fibrocartilage that resists tensional stresses, and by transversely oriented fibers, which resist the compressive stresses from the metatarsal head. It has a roughly rectangular form, being 2 to 5 mm thick. The mean length is 19 mm; the average width is 11 mm at the proximal region and 9 mm at the distal region of the second ray. Regarding biochemical structure, the plantar plate shows 75% of type I collagen and 21% of type II collagen. Collagen types III and V complete the content. The structure of the plantar plate is similar to that of the knee meniscus and the spinal annulus fibrosus, which are designed for load bearing. Besides its stabilizing and shock-absorbing functions, the plantar plate offers a gliding surface for the metatarsal head and flexor tendons. It has a strong, distal osseous attachment at the proximal phalanx plantar surface, and a thin proximal plantar attachment at the metatarsal neck. Medially and laterally, the plantar plate gives off expansions for intermetatarsal and collateral ligaments. The latter are mainly responsible for horizontal stability at MTPJ level, and are also regarded as being the most important MTPJ static vertical stabilizers.[2–5]

The tendon of the flexor digitorum longus (FDL) is attached at the base of the distal phalanx and promotes DIPJ flexion, whereas the flexor digitorum brevis (FDB) is attached at the base of the middle phalanx and promotes PIPJ flexion. There is no flexor insertion at the proximal phalanx and, as such, the plantar flexion at MTPJ level occurs because of the action of interossei and lumbricales that run beneath the axis of MTPJ. However, if the toe assumes an extended (dorsiflexed) position at the MTPJ level, those muscles become superiorly situated with regard to MTPJ level and, in this new position, lose their original flexor capability and start acting as MTPJ extensors, perpetuating the extension that pushes off inferiorly the first metatarsal head, thus increasing the pressure over the plantar plate.[6,7]

PATHOGENESIS

The exact cause of second-ray MTPJ instability is not known, but a handful of possibly predisposing factors can be seen in most cases. Plantar plate rupture usually occurs on the second ray, and the reasons possibly associated with the lesion occurring at this location include:

1. Excessive second metatarsal length with regard to the first metatarsal
2. The absence of plantar interossei and the presence of 2 dorsal interossei muscles, which may render local muscle imbalance

3. There is only one lumbrical muscle that is medially attached at the extensor apparatus at the second ray, which may also produce local muscle imbalance and create the characteristic medial deviation of the crossover deformity
4. The hallux valgus that is often associated to the lesion pushes the second toe laterally, which may lead to further instability and subluxation
5. Hypermobility with first-ray insufficiency, and lateral overload under the second ray

PATIENT HISTORY AND PHYSICAL EXAMINATION

The complaint of insidious pain associated with inadequate shoe wear is common. It is usually located at the dorsal MTPJ aspect, and/or at the plantar region at the metatarsal head.

Various grades of toe clawing (usually the second toe) are observed during standing examination. The hallux usually shows valgus deviation, lying under the second toe. The callus at the dorsal region of the PIPJ represents the friction of that region against the shoe, and at the metatarsal head the plantar region represents ray hyperpressure against the floor.

Having the patient seated, MTPJ stability is tested by the Lachman test, as described by Thompson and Hamilton.[8] The test can be graded in terms of how much proximal phalanx can vertically translate. In stage 0, there is no laxity to dorsal translation. In stage 1, the proximal phalangeal base can be subluxated, but not dislocated. In stage 2, the phalangeal base can be dislocated but also manually reduced. In stage 3, the phalangeal base is fixed in a dislocated position because of the tightness of extensor tendons, and cannot be reduced manually. The patient's pain is typically reproduced with dorsoplantar stress, and in cases of dislocation it is sometimes difficult to achieve joint reduction.

Reduction of interphalangeal joint clawing, if present, should be tested through passive mobilization.

IMAGING EXAMINATIONS

Severity of deformity is assessed by anteroposterior and lateral, standing radiograph films, and oblique views of the compromised foot. Joint congruity, metatarsal parabole, the presence of arthritic changes, and severity of deformity are all observed on radiographs. Widening of the MTPJ space can be present in early stages of joint synovitis, but the MTPJ clear space is usually reduced as the base of the proximal phalanx dorsally subluxates over the metatarsal head (**Fig. 1**).

The plantar plate itself can be studied by ultrasonography, arthrography, and magnetic resonance imaging (MRI); the latter is the examination of choice, because of its noninvasive character and its ability to show the earliest structural changes. The normal plantar plate appearance on MRI is of a smooth, curved, low-signal structure located under the metatarsal head, attaching to the base of the proximal phalanx. MRI demonstrates, especially in sagittal plane images, the lack of plate continuity at its distal attachment in the presence of a lesion.

TREATMENT OPTIONS

The treatments that have been described for MTPJ instability of lesser toes include amputation, lengthening and/or tendon transfer, periarticular soft-tissue release (capsule, collateral ligaments, and plantar plate), collateral ligament reconstruction, metatarsal shortening osteotomy, and suture of plantar plate lesion.[9–22] The

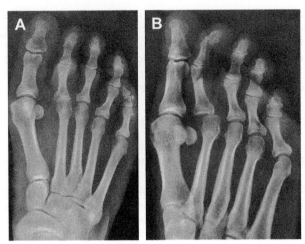

Fig. 1. (*A, B*) Anteroposterior and oblique views of the right foot, with plantar plate lesion of the second ray with joint subluxation.

combination of more than one of these procedures is often needed in the approach to treating such complex deformity.

VanderWilde and Campbell[23] reported on the results of second-toe amputations performed for chronic painful deformity, and 68% of the patients were satisfied with their results. Gallentine and DeOrio[24] published their results on removal of the second toe for severe hammertoe deformity. The study included 12 patients (17 amputations). For 11 patients the procedure met their expectation, but 8 patients observed that their hallux became more valgus after surgery. The indication for second-toe amputation is restricted to older patients with severe deformity and those who do not care about the resulting cosmetic component.

Tendon transfers do yield satisfactory results, but joint rigidity is common and often jeopardizes the final result. The most commonly used tendon transfer to stabilize MTPJ and avoid its extension is the tendon of the FDL to the extensor apparatus. Coughlin[1] recommends a flexor-to-extensor tendon transfer, performed in such a manner that the lateral limb of the FDL tendon is preferentially tightened, thus correcting the transverse malalignment. Haddad and colleagues[25] recommend extensor brevis tendon transfer for early cases of MTPJ synovitis and subluxation, and flexor-to-extensor tendon transfer for cases of toe overlap and MTPJ dislocation. In their study, 31 patients were assessed over 51.6 months of follow-up. Twenty-four patients were completely satisfied, 6 were partially satisfied, and 1 was not satisfied. Myerson and Jung[26] retrospectively assessed 59 patients who had undergone a flexor-to-extensor tendon transfer to correct MTPJ instability, with a minimum follow-up of 16 months. Weil osteotomy, PIPJ resection arthroplasty, and PIPJ fusion were the procedures additionally performed in 45%, 34%, and 13% of cases, respectively. Twenty-five patients (29 feet) were very satisfied, 15 satisfied with minor hesitancy, 6 satisfied with major hesitancy, and 14 not satisfied.[26]

A shortening osteotomy is useful for decompressing a long ray, and eventually is paramount for joint congruity reduction. Although the shortening may be performed anywhere alongside the metatarsal, Weil osteotomy, which is performed at the distal end, is more commonly used. The technique is very effective for joint decompression, although complications such as corresponding floating toe are frequent.[27]

Direct plantar plate repair can be performed through either plantar or dorsal approaches. Bouché and Heit[12] retrospectively assessed 18 patients, all of whom

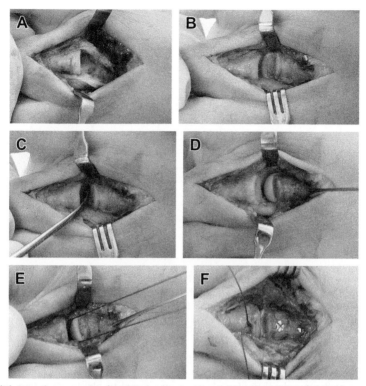

Fig. 2. (A) Dorsal approach of MTPJ demonstrating joint subluxation. (B) Weil osteotomy. (C, D) Capital fragment displaced proximal about 15 mm and provisional Kirschner-wire fixation performed to increase plantar plate lesion visualization. (E) Suture transversally passed proximal to the plantar plate lesion. (F) Final aspect, with Weil osteotomy fixated and plantar plate sutured.

were quite satisfied with the plantar repair of the plate associated to FDL tendon transfer, through a dorsal approach. A plantar plate dorsal approach associated with Weil osteotomy has been shown to be adequate for MTPJ exposure in a cadaver study.[28] Gregg and colleagues[29] retrospectively assessed the results of combined Weil osteotomy and dorsal plantar plate repair. After 26 months of follow-up, 17 of 21 patients were satisfied with the results. Weil and colleagues,[22] using a similar technique, obtained 77% of good and excellent results in 15 cases, with 22.5 months of follow-up. Coughlin and colleagues[30] have recently described a grading classification and repair of plantar plate lesion via Weil osteotomy combined with dorsally performed direct suture of plate lesion.

The proposed technique combines joint decompression by Weil osteotomy with a plantar plate repair using a pull-out technique. The second metatarsal shortening approaches the ray overload and the plantar plate suture of the lesion itself. In the authors' initial series with short-term follow-up, the results seem promising, and the incidence of floating deformity decreased compared with those cases whereby Weil osteotomy was performed without plantar plate repair.

SURGICAL TECHNIQUE

With the patient supine, under sedation and with ankle pentablock, the MTPJ is approached through a dorsal incision, and the capsule is longitudinally opened.

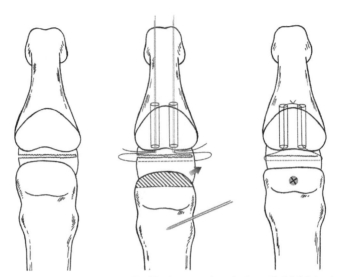

Fig. 3. Schematic of the procedure. (*Left*) Plantar plate lesion. (*Middle*) Lesion exposed through Weil osteotomy with metatarsal head retraction and sutures passing through tunnels placed onto the base of the phalanx. (*Right*) Final appearance of the repaired lesion.

Collateral ligaments can be sequentially cut to improve joint visualization. After Weil osteotomy, the metatarsal head is retracted as proximally as possible and temporarily fixated with a 1.2-mm Kirschner wire, exposing the plantar plate lesion. A 2-0 Vicryl suture is transversally applied, proximally to the lesion. Two parallel 1.5-mm holes are placed at the proximal phalanx base, from dorsal to plantar direction. A folded 1-0 steel suture is passed through each hole. The suture is brought dorsally by the steel suture and tied at the top of the proximal phalanx (**Figs. 2–4**).

POSTOPERATIVE PROTOCOL

Weight bearing with a Barouk shoe is permitted from hospital discharge until 6 weeks postoperatively. Stitches are taken out after 10 to 14 days, and active toe exercises are started from this time.

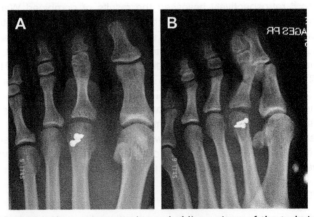

Fig. 4. (*A, B*) Postoperative anteroposterior and oblique views of the technique. Note the holes at the proximal phalanx base and the joint alignment obtained.

REFERENCES

1. Coughlin MJ. Crossover second toe deformity. Foot Ankle 1987;8(1):29–39.
2. Johnston RB, Smith J, Daniels T. The plantar plate of the lesser toes: an anatomical study in human cadavers. Foot Ankle Int 1994;15(5):276–82.
3. Deland JT, Lee KT, Sobel M, et al. Anatomy of the plantar plate and its attachments in the lesser metatarsal phalangeal joint. Foot Ankle Int 1995;16(8):480–6.
4. Bhatia D, Myerson MS, Curtis MJ, et al. Anatomical restraints to dislocation of the second metatarsophalangeal joint and assessment of a repair technique. J Bone Joint Surg Am 1994;76:1371–5.
5. Sarrafian SK. Retaining systems and compartments. In: Anatomy of the foot and ankle. Philadelphia: JB Lippincott; 1993. p. 142–57.
6. Myerson MS, Shereff MJ. The pathological anatomy of claw and hammer toes. J Bone Joint Surg Am 1989;71:45–9.
7. Marks RM. Anatomy and pathophysiology of lesser toe deformities. In: Richardson EG, Myerson MS, editors. Foot ankle clinics: lesser toe deformities. Philadelphia, PA: W.B. Saunders; 1998. p. 199–214, 3–3.
8. Thompson FM, Hamilton WG. Problems of the second metatarsophalangeal joint. Orthopedics 1987;10(1):83–9.
9. Barca F, Acciaro AL. Surgical correction of crossover deformity of the second toe: a technique for tenodesis. Foot Ankle Int 2004;25(9):620–4.
10. Blitz NM, Ford LA, Christensen JC. Plantar plate repair of the second metatarsophalangeal joint: technique and tips. J Foot Ankle Surg 2004;43(4):266–70.
11. Bogy LT, Vranes R, Goforth WP, et al. Correction of overlapping second toe deformity: long-term results including a 7-year follow-up. J Foot Surg 1992;31(4):319–23.
12. Bouché RT, Heit EJ. Combined plantar plate and hammertoe repair with flexor digitorum longus tendon transfer for chronic, severe sagittal plane instability of the lesser metatarsophalangeal joints: preliminary observations. J Foot Ankle Surg 2008;47(2):125–37.
13. Ford LA, Collins KB, Christensen JC. Stabilization of the subluxed second metatarsophalangeal joint: flexor tendon transfer versus primary repair of the plantar plate. J Foot Ankle Surg 1998;37(3):217–22.
14. Gazdaga A, Cracchiolo A. Surgical treatment of patients with painful instability of the second metatarsophalangeal joint. Foot Ankle Int 1998;19(3):137–43.
15. Graziano TA. Correction of crossover second toe deformity. Clin Podiatr Med Surg 1996;13(2):269–78.
16. Johnson A, Aibinder W, Deland JT. Clinical tip: partial plantar plate release for correction of crossover second toe. Foot Ankle Int 2008;29(11):1145–7.
17. Johnson JB, Price TW. Crossover second toe deformity: etiology and treatment. J Foot Surg 1989;28(5):417–20.
18. Lui TH, Chan KB. Technique tip: modified extensor digitorum brevis tendon transfer for crossover second toe correction. Foot Ankle Int 2007;28(4):521–3.
19. Lui TH. Correction of crossover deformity of second toe by combined plantar plate tenodesis and extensor digitorum brevis transfer: a minimally invasive approach. Arch Orthop Trauma Surg 2011;131(9):1247–52.
20. Sampath JS, Barrie JL. Results of flexor-to-extensor and extensor brevis tendon transfer for correction of the crossover second toe deformity. Foot Ankle Int 2000;21(10):872.
21. Thompson FM, Deland JT. Flexor tendon transfer for metatarsophalangeal instability of the second toe. Foot Ankle 1993;14(7):385–8.

22. Weil L, Sung W, Weil LS, et al. Anatomic plantar plate repair using the Weil meta-tarsal osteotomy approach. Foot Ankle Spec 2011;4(3):145–50.
23. VanderWilde R, Campbell D. Second toe amputation for chronic painful deformity. Conference at the 23rd Annual Meeting of the American Orthopaedic Foot & Ankle Society. San Francisco (CA): Calif; 1993.
24. Gallentine JW, DeOrio JK. Removal of the second toe for severe hammertoe deformity in elderly patients. Foot Ankle Int 2005;26(5):353–8.
25. Haddad SL, Sabbagh RC, Resch S, et al. Results of flexor-to-extensor and extensor brevis tendon transfer for correction of the crossover second toe defor-mity. Foot Ankle Int 1999;20(12):781–8.
26. Myerson MS, Jung HG. The role of toe flexor-to-extensor transfer in correcting metatarsophalangeal joint instability of the second toe. Foot Ankle Int 2005; 26(9):675–9.
27. Migues A, Slullitel G, Bilbao F, et al. Floating-toe deformity as a complication of the Weil osteotomy. Foot Ankle Int 2004;25(9):609–13.
28. Cooper MT, Coughlin MJ. Sequential dissection for exposure of the second meta-tarsophalangeal joint. Foot Ankle Int 2011;32(3):294–9.
29. Gregg J, Silberstein M, Clark C, et al. Plantar plate repair and Weil osteotomy for metatarsophalangeal joint instability. Foot Ankle Surg 2007;13(3):116–21.
30. Coughlin MJ, Baumfeld DS, Nery C. Second MTP joint instability: grading of the deformity and description of surgical repair of capsular insufficiency. Phys Sportsmed 2011;39(3):132–41.

Peroneus Longus Transfer for Drop Foot in Hansen Disease

Jose Carlos Cohen, MD[a],*, Elifaz de Freitas Cabral, MD[b]

KEYWORDS

- Peroneus longus transfer • Drop foot • Hansen disease

KEY POINTS

- Nerve injury is a central feature of the pathogenesis of leprosy because of the unique tendency of *Mycobacterium leprae* to invade Schwann cells and the peripheral nervous system, causing a mononeuritis multiplex of immunologic origin that results in autonomic, sensory, and motor neuropathy.
- Early diagnosis of leprosy, along with early detection and treatment of neuropathy, are the means to prevent permanent primary impairments.[1]
- Investigators state that up to about 4 to 5 skin lesions constitutes paucibacillary leprosy, whereas about 5 or more constitutes multibacillary leprosy.

INTRODUCTION

Leprosy, or Hansen disease, is a chronic infectious disease caused by *Mycobacterium leprae*. The skin and nervous manifestations of the disease present a singular clinical picture that is easily recognized. After India, Brazil is the country with the greatest number of cases in the world.[2] Nerve injury is a central feature of the pathogenesis of leprosy because of the unique tendency of *M leprae* to invade Schwann cells and the peripheral nervous system, causing a mononeuritis multiplex of immunologic origin that results in autonomic, sensory, and motor neuropathy. Early diagnosis of leprosy, along with early detection and treatment of neuropathy, are the means to prevent permanent primary impairments.[1]

The World Health Organization (WHO) classification system is used to differentiate the 2 clinical presentations of leprosy. The 2009 WHO classifications are based on the number of bacilli per skin lesions, as follows: paucibacillary leprosy, skin lesions with no bacilli (*M leprae*) seen in a skin smear; multibacillary leprosy, skin lesions with bacilli (*M leprae*) seen in a skin smear.

---

[a] Foot and Ankle Service, Department of Orthopaedic Surgery, Federal University Hospital of Rio de Janeiro-UFRJ, Rua Alberto de Campos 172 apartment 101, Ipanema, CEP 22411-030, Rio de Janeiro, Brazil; [b] Rua Alexandre Guimarães, 1927, Areal - Porto Velho, Rondonia, CEP 76.804-373, Brazil
* Corresponding author.
E-mail address: cohenorto@yahoo.com

Foot Ankle Clin N Am 17 (2012) 425–436
http://dx.doi.org/10.1016/j.fcl.2012.06.005
1083-7515/12/$ – see front matter © 2012 Elsevier Inc. All rights reserved.

However, the WHO further modifies these 2 classifications with clinical criteria because of the nonavailability or nondependability of skin-smear services. The clinical system of classification for the purpose of treatment includes the use of number of skin lesions and/or one or no nerve involved as the basis for grouping patients with leprosy into multibacillary and paucibacillary leprosy. Investigators state that up to about 4 to 5 skin lesions constitutes paucibacillary leprosy, whereas about 5 or more constitutes multibacillary leprosy.

The irreversible motor, sensory, and autonomic impairments caused by leprosy lead to increasing secondary impairments long after the disease process has been arrested. The progressive physical impairments caused by the disease process are compounded by the psychological and social consequences that adversely influence the participation in society of those affected.[3]

INDICATIONS AND CONTRAINDICATIONS

One of the most common secondary disabilities caused by Hansen disease is drop foot, which is found in 2% to 5% of newly diagnosed patients with leprosy.[4] Leprosy neuritis affects nerves where they are close to the skin and pass through a narrow fibro-osseus canal. In the leg, this includes the involvement of the common peroneal nerve at the neck of the fibula, which leads to foot drop, and the posterior tibial nerve in the tarsal tunnel, which produces anesthesia of the sole. When both nerves are damaged, the main impact of walking is on the anesthetic forefoot rather than on the heel and causes trophic ulceration. Unlike the clinical picture of traumatic injury of the common peroneal nerve, in which both of its branches (the deep peroneal nerve and the superficial peroneal nerve) are involved, in leprosy there is the possibility of isolated involvement of the deep peroneal nerve branch, sparing the superficial peroneal branch. The classic clinical manifestation of supinated equino varus deformity associated with injury of the common peroneal nerve commonly seen after a traumatic injury, caused by overpull of plantar flexors and inverters powered by the intact tibial nerve and loss of dorsiflexors and evertors powered by the compromised common peroneal nerve, is replaced by a selective paralysis of the anterior compartment of the leg with preservation of function of both peroneal tendons in the lateral compartment. In addition, the peroneus longus can overpower the weak anterior tibial tendon (its antagonist on the first metatarsal), and produces marked plantar flexion in the first metatarsal that can cause secondary varus in the hindfoot.

The result is a well-balanced foot, regarding the inversion and eversion moments of forces, because both tibialis posterior and peroneal brevis tendons are intact. Although many investigators still recommend the tibialis posterior tendon transfer even when there is normal function of the peroneal tendons, we do not think it is necessary to sacrifice a major tendon stabilizer of the arch of the foot in these selected cases.

The occurrence of flatfoot after harvesting the posterior tibial tendon for drop foot in which both the anterior and lateral compartments of the leg are paralyzed is rare in the literature, and this may be because, in the palsied foot, loss of peroneus brevis function (as a result of nerve injury) and loss of posterior tibial tendon (as a result of tendon transfer) result in a new dynamic balance,[5] preventing the arch breakdown. In contrast, in the presence of normal function of the superficial peroneal nerve, the primary evertor of the foot, the peroneus brevis muscle, is unopposed after the posterior tibial tendon (PTT) transfer, leading to a higher possibility of development of flatfoot, because the deforming force exerted by the peroneus brevis is a well-recognized feature in the development of adult acquired flatfoot, leading to hindfoot valgus and midfoot collapse caused by insufficiency of the posterior tibial tendon.[6]

Yeap and colleagues[7] reported on the results of 12 patients undergoing posterior tibial tendon transfer through the interosseus membrane in patients without leprosy, and found 4 patients with some flattening of the medial longitudinal arch. In addition, the use of the anterior transfer of the tibialis posterior tendon in cerebral palsy to treat spastic equinovarus has led to collapse of the talonavicular joint with significant calcaneus and valgus deformities of the foot in children.[8,9]

To prevent this complication, Klaue and colleagues[10] recommended the simultaneous transfer of the flexor digitorum longus to the medial cuneiform during the PTT transfer in cases of posttraumatic drop foot, pes equinus, and cerebral palsy to restore dorsiflexion.

The objectives of tendon transfer for treatment of drop foot are to improve functional deficit by restoring or reinforcing lost functions, to neutralize deforming forces, and to gain stability, eliminating the need for bracing during gait.[2,5]

The correction of drop foot in leprosy with PTT transfer is well established in the literature, although there is still some debate concerning the need to use the interosseus route. Srinivasan and colleagues[11] recommend the anterior transposition of the PTT subcutaneously, dividing the tendon into 2 slips and suturing the medial slip to the extensor hallucis longus (EHL) and the lateral slip to the extensor digitorum longus (EDL). Advocates for the circumtibial (CT; ie, subcutaneous) transfer claim that is unnecessary to use the interosseus route, because the CT transfer is easier and safer to perform, there is no risk of injury or tethering of the neurovascular bundle, the tendon is allowed to glide smoothly, and it diminishes the possibility of adhesions of the tendon or muscle belly in the interosseous (IO) membrane. In contrast, advocates for the IO transfer claim advantages such as the direct pull of the tendon, producing less inversion deformity, and the possibility of a greater length of tendon for insertion, thus preventing the tenodesis effect related to an overly high tension of the suture transfer. Hall[12] reported that the subcutaneous route gave greater dorsiflexion (25°–30° compared with only 17°) than the interosseus route, but Soares,[4] in a long-term study comparing PTT transfer using the CT route with the IO route for drop foot in patients with leprosy, reported an unacceptably high rate of recurrent inversion in the CT group even in those cases with the peroneal tendons intact, leading to ulceration of the lateral border of the foot, and recommended that the CT route should be reserved for patients with a calcified and unyielding IO membrane. He also reported better active dorsiflexion in the IO group, although there was less active plantar flexion than with the CT route.

Another controversial issue is the point of reinsertion of the tendon, which varies according to the foot deformity present. In a cadaver study,[13] comparing the CT and IO routes for PTT transfer to the dorsum of the foot, in which the insertion sites were tested separately for the medial, intermediate and lateral cuneiform, and the cuboid, concluded that the optimal insertion site for PTT transfer to produce maximal dorsiflexion with minimal pronation was the IO route, with the insertion site in the lateral cuneiform.

The necessity for bone fixation instead of tendon-to-tendon reattachment is also debatable. Tendon-to-tendon suture addresses the difficulties related to tendon-to-bone procedures and donor tendon length. It allows the surgeon to adjust and modulate tendon tension, appropriately verifying foot posture before suturing is completed .Bone fixation provides a stronger attachment site and theoretically prevents the stretching that might occur over time when a tendon-to-tendon transfer is performed. However, the occurrence of a Charcot arthropathy as a consequence of a creation of a bone tunnel in patients with leprosy is possible.[14–16] Some investigators state that the presence of leprosy is a contraindication for bone fixation, and that all those cases should be managed with tendon-to-tendon procedures. Warren[16] in 1968 advised against bone fixation in correction of foot drop in leprosy, because "it has been assumed that surgical intervention with the tarsal bones must increase the tendency to bone breakdown after surgery." Our recommendation is that, in paucibacillary cases, the transfer should be to bone, and, in multibacillary cases, we do not recommend bone fixation because of the risk of Charcot arthropathy, anchoring the tendon to soft tissues in the dorsum of the foot.

Carayon and colleagues[17] use both the PTT and the flexor digitorum longus (FDL) through the interosseus membrane with tendon-to-tendon insertion, in which the PTT is sutured to the tibialis anterior and the FDL to both the tendons of EHL and EDL. They reported 31 cases, of which 26 cases were drop foot caused by Hansen disease. The results were excellent in 11 (active dorsiflexion of 15° or more and active plantar flexion of more than 30°), good in 6 (active dorsiflexion of 5°–10° and active plantar flexion of 15°–20°, fair in 2 (no active dorsiflexion but correction of drop foot and plantar flexion to 10°), and poor in 3 (the foot held in a disabling degree of plantar flexion and no dorsiflexion). In an analysis of the fair and poor results, they noted that most failures were caused by loss of tension in the transferred tendons at the point of fixation, which is one of the problems with tendon-to-tendon fixation.

The use of the peroneal longus tendon as the single dorsiflexor of the foot in leprosy was first reported by Srinivasan and colleagues,[11] who wrote that "with the peronei tendons intact, removal of the tibial posterior from the medial side of the ankle might cause instability of the foot." This method has the advantage of leaving the PTT intact on the medial side, whereas the peroneus brevis was left to balance it on the lateral side. They also stated that, if the patient later developed paralysis of the peroneals, the tibialis posterior could still be used as a motor. In his original technique, he split the tendon into 2 halves and performed a tendon-to-tendon transfer into the EHL, EDL, and peroneus tertius. In our surgical procedure, we use the entire tendon, use a subcutaneous route, and anchor it to the intermediate cuneiforme with a drill hole or to the intercuneiform ligaments. Two benefits are derived from this tendon transfer. A deforming force (plantar flexion of the first metatarsal producing forefoot-driven hindfoot varus) is eliminated, because there is an unopposed pull of the peroneus longus against the weak tibialis anterior tendon, and a correcting force (dorsiflexion in the ankle) is established. Morton[18] pointed out that the peroneus longus had been a lateral dorsiflexor in early evolutionary stages, justifying its use as a dorsiflexor muscle.

The bridle procedure was described by Riordan and later modified by Rodriguez.[19] It also uses the peroneus longus tendon, combining the transfer of the peroneus longus with the PTT[19] to balance the foot in dorsiflexion. However, in this surgery the peroneus longus is not used as the primarily active dorsiflexor, because it is divided proximally, rerouted anteriorly to the lateral malleolus, and anastomosed with the anterior and posterior tibialis tendons in the anterior leg.

Despite the peroneus longus transfer for drop foot being described more than 40 years ago, there is still some question of its efficacy. Sigvard Hansen[20] stated in his textbook that, "transfer of the peroneus longus seems to violate too many rules to be effective. In this procedure, the peroneus longus is removed from its normal bed, carried a long distance, and expected to go from plantar flexion in stance phase to dorsiflexion in swing phase."

In addition, the peroneus longus transfer alone may not be as strong as the tibialis posterior. **Tables 1** and **2** show the different moments of rotation of the extrinsic tendons around the ankle and subtalar joints, and show that the tibialis posterior and peroneus longus tendons have similar amounts of force.

When using the PTT as an active dorsiflexor, the tendon transfer should act partially as a tenodesis, producing a decreased range of motion in the plantar direction. After

Table 1
Moments of rotation of the extrinsic tendons in relation to the ankle joint

Tendon	Moment of Rotation (Nm)
Flexor Tendons	
Achilles tendon	164
Flexor digitorum longus	3.9
Tibialis posterior	3.9
Peroneus longus	3.9
Peroneus brevis	2.9
Flexor hallucis longus	8.8
Extensor Tendons	
Tibialis anterior	25
Extensor hallucis longus	3.9
Extensor digitorum longus	7.8
Peroneus tertius	4.9

Data from Sarrafian SK. Anatomy of the foot and ankle. 2nd edition. Philadelphia: Lippincott; 1993.

bridle PTT for drop foot, Gellman and colleagues[21] reported an average ankle dorsiflexion of 10° and plantar flexion most commonly measuring 0°. The subtalar joint range of motion was significantly reduced to 0% to 25% of the nonoperative side.

Because it is not necessary to reroute the peroneus longus tendon through the interosseus membrane, a better excursion of the tendon is possible, avoiding the tenodesis effect related to adhesions in the IO space. This option potentially increases the range of motion after the tendon transfer. However, according to biomechanical principles of tendon transfers, when a stance-phase muscle (both the posterior tendon and peroneus longus are stance-phase muscles) is converted to a swing-phase muscle (nonphasic transfer), there is a chance that it will function more as a tenodesis than as an active muscle transfer, regardless of the route used for the transfer.

Table 2
Moments of rotation of the extrinsic tendons in relation to the foot plate and the subtalar joint axis

Tendon	Moment of Rotation (Nm)
Supinator Tendons	
Achilles tendon	48
Flexor digitorum longus	7.8
Tibialis anterior	9.8
Tibialis posterior	18
Flexor hallucis longus	7.8
Pronator Tendons	
Peroneus longus	17
Peroneus brevis	13
Extensor digitorum longus	7.8
Peroneus tertius	4.9
Extensor hallucis longus	1
Tibialis anterior	2.9

Data from Sarrafian SK. Anatomy of the foot and ankle. 2nd edition. Philadelphia: Lippincott; 1993.

PREOPERATIVE PLANNING

It is of paramount importance that the disease process is controlled and the patient is adequately treated with multidrug therapy. In addition, it must be established that there has been at least 1 year without inflammatory reactions (reverse reaction or erythema nodosum). This is because the surgical procedure itself might cause those reactions, compromising the surgical results. The neurologic damage must be irreversible, which is considered after 1 year without improvement of the motor function or established earlier with eletroneuromuscular studies. Equinus contracture of the Achilles tendon must be tested for. Patients with passive dorsiflexion of less than 20° should have percutaneous lengthening of the Achilles at the same time as the transfer. It may be advisable to perform percutaneous lengthening in all patients, because the more powerful Achilles tendon will eventually overcome the weaker peroneus longus. The ideal patient for the peroneus longus transfer has normal motor strength in the peroneus longus muscle, but motor strength of +4/+5 is also acceptable and provides enough power for ambulation out of a brace. As in all tendon transfers, any fixed joint deformities must be corrected to gain a successful result, requiring arthrodesis, osteotomy, or soft tissue releases. The presence of clawing of the toes should be noted and treated if necessary.

We always instruct our patients how to contract the tendon to be transferred in an isolated manner in the preoperative period to maximize our results. Factors such as motivation, self-care, and whether the patient is capable of following the postoperative recommendation are important issues.

SURGICAL TECHNIQUE

With the patient lying supine on the operating table, a pneumatic tourniquet is applied to the thigh. The entire lower limb is prepped and draped in a regular fashion. If the limb is overly externally rotated, an ipsilateral bump is place under the buttock to internally rotate the leg. Patients are given preoperative intravenous antibiotics (**Fig. 1**). This procedure may be performed with the patient under spinal, epidural, or general anesthesia. Testing for equinus contracture is performed. If present, a percutaneous lengthening of the Achilles is done. The peroneal tendons are accessed through a short incision at the level of the base of the fifth metatarsal directed approximately 3 cm toward the lateral malleolus, parallel to the peroneus longus tendon. The dissection is carried down to the level of the paratenon. The sural nerve usually runs more cranially; if identified, it is retracted. The peroneal tendon sheath is then opened and the peroneus

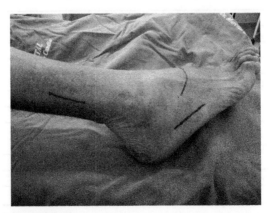

Fig. 1. Marking of skin incisions.

longus can typically be seen beneath the peroneus brevis. The peroneus longus is pulled using an elevator and secured by a suture.[22] Before cutting the tendon, it is important to tenodese the distal stump of the peroneus longus with the peroneus brevis tendon using a side-by-side suture (Ethbond no. 2; **Fig. 2**), which prevents elevation of the first metatarsal (dorsal bunion) because of the unopposed pull of the tibialis anterior tendon (although this tendon is theoretically weak in drop foot, I always tenodese the distal stump of the peroneus longus to the peroneus brevis tendon). Now the peroneus longus tendon can be sectioned as distally as possible in the cuboid tunnel and the proximal stump tagged with a whipstitch suture. A second incision is then made proximally on the lateral compartment in the distal third of the leg, about 8 cm proximal to the tip of the fibula at the level of the musculotendinous junction of the peroneus longus. Protect the superficial peroneal nerve. The tendon sheath of the peroneus longus is incised and the peroneus longus tendon is identified and pulled proximally in the wound (**Fig. 3**). The tendon is kept moist with a sponge or allowed to remain in its sheath during dissection of the dorsal tarsus. A third 3-cm transverse incision is made on the dorsum of the foot over the intermediate cuneiform (**Fig. 4**). Care is taken with the superficial peroneal nerve and extensor tendons. Protect the deep neurovascular bundle, which is usually encountered in this approach; it is directly deep to the muscle of the extensor hallucis brevis. Identify the intermediate cuneiform, leaving the periosteum and capsular tissue intact. A tunnelization clamp is passed subcutaneously from this incision to the proximal lateral wound and the tagged peroneal longus tendon is delivered distally (**Fig. 5**). Using a fluoroscopic image is helpful to confirm the position for creation of the bone tunnel in the intermediate cuneiform. The bone tunnel is made from dorsal to plantar using drill bits and curettes as necessary to accommodate the tendon. A straight Keith needle is used to pass the tag suture through the bone tunnel, exiting the sole of the foot. The foot is then held in maximal dorsiflexion (if possible, in 30° of dorsiflexion) and the tag suture in the plantar aspect of the foot should be pulled distally, thereby pulling the tendon end into the tunnel. The proximal stump of the peroneus longus is then fixed to the bone tunnel using staples, biotenodesis screws, or anchors. If possible, we augment the anchor point with several nonabsorbable sutures from the periosteum surrounding the tunnel to the tendon directly at the entrance of the tunnel. In multibacillary cases, we avoid using the bone insertion because of the potential for Charcot arthropathy. In these situation, we insert the peroneus longus transfer in the lateral margin of the intertarsal ligaments (**Fig. 6**).

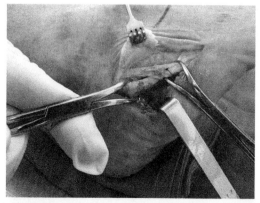

Fig. 2. Tenodesis of the distal stump of the peroneus longus to the peroneus brevis before cutting the tendon.

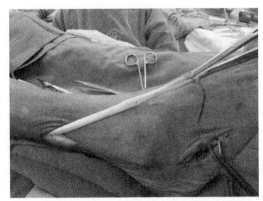

Fig. 3. Delivery of the peroneus longus tendon through the lateral incision in the lower leg.

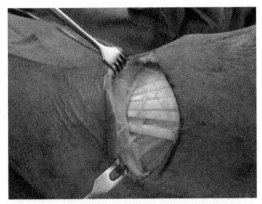

Fig. 4. Third incision over the dorsum of the foot, exposing the extensor tendons and taking care with the neurovascular structures.

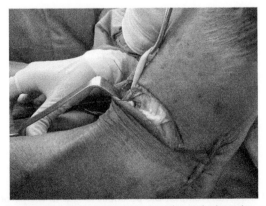

Fig. 5. After rerouting the peroneus longus tendon through the subcutaneous route.

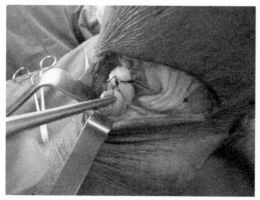

Fig. 6. Suture of the peroneus longus tendon to the intertarsal ligaments with nonabsorbable stitches.

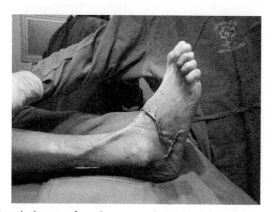

Fig. 7. Wounds closed, the transferred peroneus longus can be seen under the skin.

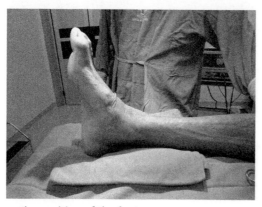

Fig. 8. Final postoperative position of the foot.

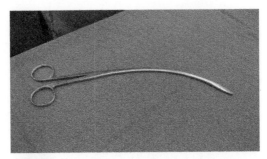

Fig. 9. Tunnelization clamp.

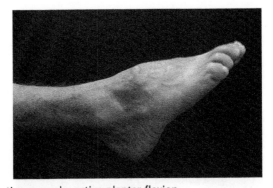

Fig. 10. Postoperative example: active plantar flexion.

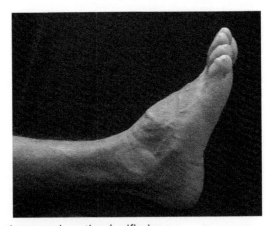

Fig. 11. Postoperative example: active dorsiflexion.

The wound is irrigated and closed in a regular fashion. At the end of the procedure, the foot should rest in 20° to 25° of dorsiflexion and a well-padded short leg cast is applied, also holding the foot in the desired dorsiflexion position (**Figs. 7–11**).

POSTOPERATIVE MANAGEMENT

The cast is maintained for 2 weeks. The cast is then removed and stitches taken out. The patient is then placed in a weight-bearing cast and is allowed partial weight bearing with use of crutches. Six weeks after the procedure, the cast is removed and the patient is instructed to ambulate in an ankle-foot orthosis brace or walker boot. At 8 weeks, the rehabilitation program to improve strengthening, proprioception, gait, and range of motion is started, but the protected ambulation is continued for 4 months. In addition, the patient should use a cam boot for sleeping until 4 months after surgery. Physical therapy is beneficial to train the peroneus longus in its new phase, and the patient is encouraged to walk as much as possible. If the muscle fails to adapt to its new function, electrical stimulation should be added to the physical therapy program.

RESULTS

From 1998 to 2008, we operated on 57 cases of drop foot caused by Hansen disease, with 61 feet, 59% men and 41% women, with an average age of 39 years. Among these, 19 cases were considered to have a selective paralysis of the anterior compartment of the leg, with functioning peroneal tendons. The postoperative results showed that average dorsiflexion was 10° and plantar flexion was 32°. Fifteen cases were very satisfied with the procedure, being able to walk without any kind of supportive brace. Two cases were satisfied with the result, but still wear a brace for walking long distances. We had 2 poor results, with weak dorsiflexion after the transfer. These cases may not have been good candidates for the procedure because of undetected weakness of the peroneal tendons.

POSSIBLE CONCERNS, INDICATIONS, AND FUTURE OF THE TECHNIQUE

We are concerned that the peroneus longus transfer for drop foot might result in varus deformity of the hindfoot in the middle to long term, because the remaining force provided by the peroneus brevis may not be enough to counteract the powerful pull of the tibialis posterior tendon. Other possible indications for the peroneus longus transfer are posttraumatic anterior or anterior and deep posterior compartment syndromes. Both of these conditions are characterized by drop-foot deformity and absence of anterior tibial tendon function.

REFERENCES

1. Van Brakel WH. Peripheral neuropathy in leprosy and its consequences. Lepr Rev 2000;71(Suppl):S146–53.
2. Araujo MA. Leprosy in Brazil. Rev Soc Bras Med Trop 2003;36(3) [in Portuguese].
3. Smith WC. Review of current research in prevention of nerve damage in leprosy. Lepr Rev 2000;71(Suppl):s138–44 [discussion: S145].
4. Soares D. Tibialis posterior transfer for the correction of foot drop in leprosy. Long term outcome. J Bone Joint Surg Br 1996;78(1):61–2.
5. Vigasio A, Marcoccio I, Patelli A, et al. New tendon transfer for correction of drop-foot in common peroneal nerve palsy. Clin Orthop Relat Res 2008;466:1454–66.

6. Mizel MS, Temple HT, Scranton PE, et al. Role of the peroneal tendons in the production of the deformed foot with posterior tibial tendon deficiency. Foot Ankle Int 1999;20(5):285–9.

7. Yeap JS, Birch R, Singh D. Long-term results of tibialis posterior tendon transfer for drop-foot. Int Orthop 2001;25:114–8.

8. Turner JW, Cooper RR. Anterior transfer of the tibialis posterior through the interosseus membrane. Clin Orthop Relat Res 1972;83:241–4.

9. Schneider M, Balon K. Deformity of the foot following anterior transfer of the posterior tibial tendon and lengthening of the Achilles tendon for spastic equinovarus. Clin Orthop Relat Res 1977;(125):113–8.

10. Klaue K, Fandler JP, Speck M, et al. Tendon Transfers. In: Wulker N, Stephens MM, Cracchilo A III, editors. An atlas of foot and ankle surgery. 2nd edition. Taylor & Francis; 2005. p. 199–215.

11. Srinivasan H, Mukherjee SM, Subramaniam RA. Two-tailed transfer of tibialis posterior for correction of drop-foot in leprosy. J Bone Joint Surg Br 1968;50(3): 623–8.

12. Hall G. A review of drop-foot corrective surgery. Lepr Rev 1977;48:185–92.

13. Goh JC, Lee PY, Lee EH, et al. Biomechanical study on tibialis posterior tendon transfers. Clin Orthop Relat Res 1995;(319):297–302.

14. Anderson JG. Foot drop in leprosy. Lepr Rev 1964;35:41–6.

15. Harris JR, Brand PW. Patterns of disintegration of the tarsus in the anaesthetic foot. J Bone Joint Surg Br 1966;48:4–16.

16. Warren AG. The correction of foot drop in leprosy. J Bone Joint Surg Br 1968;50: 629–34.

17. Carayon A, Bourrel P, Bourges M, et al. Dual transfer of the posterior tibial and flexor digitorum longus tendons for drop-foot: report of thirty-one cases. J Bone Joint Surg Am 1967;49(1):144–8.

18. Morton DJ. The human foot: its evolution, physiology, and functional disorders. Morningside Heights (New York): Columbia University Press; 1935.

19. Rodriguez RP. The bridle procedure in the treatment of paralysis of the foot. Foot Ankle 1992;13(2):63–9.

20. Hansen ST Jr. Functional reconstruction of the foot and ankle. Philadelphia: Lippincott Williams & Wilkins; 2000.

21. Gellman RE, Anderson RD, Davis WH. Master techniques in orthopaedic surgery. The foot and ankle. 2nd edition. Philadelphia: Lippincott Williams & Wilkins; 2002. p. 597–613.

22. Kilger R, Knupp M, Hintermann B. Peroneus longus to peroneus brevis tendon transfer. Tech Foot Ankle Surg 2009;8(3):146–9.

Calcaneonavicular Ligament
Anatomy, Diagnosis, and Treatment

Alberto Macklin Vadell, MD, Marcela Peratta, MD*

KEYWORDS

- Spring ligament • Calcaneonavicular complex • Adult flat foot
- Posterior tibial tendon dysfunction

KEY POINTS

- The calcaneonavicular ligament is a recently recognized structure between the navicular and the calcaneal, composed mainly of 2 bundles, the superomedial and inferoplantar.
- The ligament complex has static function and distinctive of histologic composition and vascularization.
- Rupture of the spring ligament may be isolated or associated with posterior tibial tendon disorders; the clinical presentation of the lesion is unclear and may mimic a posterior tibial tendon dysfunction.

INTRODUCTION

Wrongly called the spring ligament, the calcaneonavicular ligament has recently been identified. Its anatomic description, disorders, diagnosis, and treatment are still uncertain and controversial. The calcaneonavicular ligament injury may be single or related to varying degrees of posterior tibial tendon lesion. This article focuses on its anatomic description, and suitable diagnostic and reconstruction methods.

ANATOMY

The calcaneonavicular ligament complex includes the ligaments between the calcaneal and the navicular in the superomedial and inferoplantar region (**Fig. 1**). The calcaneonavicular or spring ligament is classically described with 2 bundles, superomedial and inferior. However, besides these 2 components, a third structure was identified, called the midplantar oblique ligament,[1,2] which is not always present and is difficult to recognize.[3]

The superomedial bundle originates in the sustentaculum tali and the anterior edge of the anterior facet of the calcaneus, sharing the attachment with the tibiocalcaneal fibers of the superficial deltoid ligament (**Fig. 2**); it fans out distally to form the floor of the posterior tibial tendon and attaches to the superomedial and inferior edge of

Cerviño Av. 4679, 2nd floor, 1426 Buenos Aires, Argentina
* Corresponding author.
E-mail address: marcelaperatta@gmail.com

Foot Ankle Clin N Am 17 (2012) 437–448
http://dx.doi.org/10.1016/j.fcl.2012.07.002
1083-7515/12/$ – see front matter © 2012 Elsevier Inc. All rights reserved.

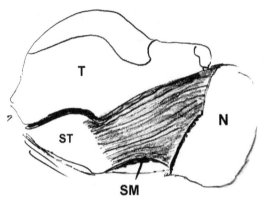

Fig. 1. Superomedial ligament (SM, superomedial; T, talus; N, navicular; ST, sustentaculum tali).

the navicular, sharing the attachment with the posterior tibial tendon (**Figs. 3** and **4**).[4] It is the most frequently found bundle in posterior tibial tendon surgeries, and where the usual lesions are located. The inferoplantar bundle originates in the coronoid fossa of the calcaneus, in the anterior aspect of the sustentaculum tali, and attaches to the inferior surface of the navicular (**Fig. 5**A, B).[5]

There is no consensus on the anatomic description of the calcaneonavicular ligament. Sarrafian[6] describes two separate structures: one is wide and articular, in contact with the deltoid ligament, and the other is inferior and plantar, which he considers to be the true spring ligament and to correspond with the lower portion of the head of the talus. McMinn and Hutchings identify the calcaneonavicular ligament as the superomedial structure and make no reference to the plantar portion. Davis and colleagues[7] found 2 separate ligaments that together form the acetabulum pedis. Numerous histologic studies have shown the absence of elastin[8] or elastic fibers[9] in the calcaneo-navicular ligament complex, thus the ligament lacks elastic properties (**Fig. 6**) and therefore spring ligament is not a suitable name.

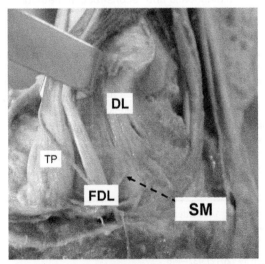

Fig. 2. Anatomical relantioships (DL, deltoid ligament; TP, posterior tibialis tendon; FDL, flexor digitorum longus; SM, superomedial ligament).

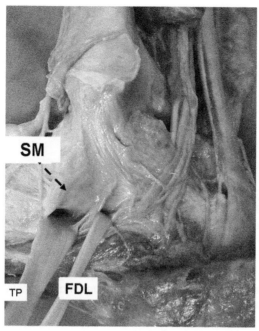

Fig. 3. Anatomical relantionships (SM, superomedial ligament; TP, posterior tibialis tendon; FDL, flexor digitorum longus).

However, the superomedial bundle is dorsally covered by fibrocartilage,[2] turning it into the strongest and broadest of the three structures. The fibrocartilage would also suggests that the ligament is subject to compression and stress at the level of the talo-navicular joint. According to Davis and colleagues,[7] the major blood supply to the superomedial bundle comes from its proximal and distal bony attachments. The proximal supply originates in the calcaneal branches of the medial plantar artery and supplies the proximal and plantar third, whereas the scaphoid branches of the medial plantar artery supply the distal and plantar third, and the dorsal and central third of the bundle are avascular. This finding was confirmed by Davis and colleagues[7] and by Macklin and colleagues[9] in specimens without tissue necrosis in which the absence

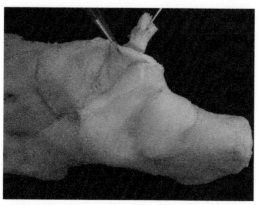

Fig. 4. Dorsal view of the foot (without talus) Superomedial ligament held by the clamp.

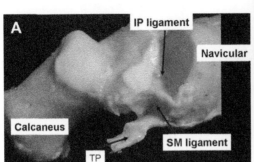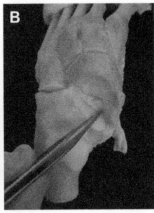

Fig. 5. (*A*) Dorsal view (without talus) IP inferoplantar ligament, SM superomedial ligament, TP posterior tibialis tendon. (*B*) Dorsal view (without talus) inferoplantar ligament held by the clamp.

of central vascularity in the fibrochondral region was shown, as well as the presence of arterioles, veins, and capillaries in the areas surrounding the fibrochondroid core (**Figs. 7–10**); this arrangement would prevent repairs to a lesion in the area.[7]

FUNCTION

The calcaneonavicular ligament complex, together with the anterior and middle facets of the calcaneus and the proximal surface of the navicular, form the acetabulum pedis. This ligament complex has two functions: (1) it is the static support of the head of the talus and provides stability to the talonavicular joint, and (2) it provides the medial longitudinal arch support.[3] Moreover, the calcaneonavicular, deltoid, and plantar ligaments, and the plantar fascia passively, together with the posterior tibial tendon actively, stabilize the subtalar and talonavicular joints.

SPRING LIGAMENT TEARS: CLINICAL PRESENTATION

The clinical presentation of the single calcaneonavicular ligament lesion varies; it is essential to consider this disorder when evaluating a patient with a painful posterior

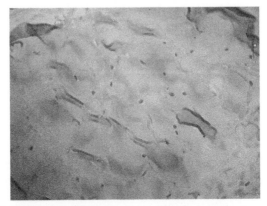

Fig. 6. Absence of elastic fibers (histological cut of SM ligament).

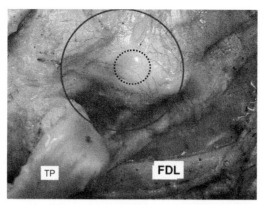

Fig. 7. SM ligament with chinese ink. Periferic area with vascularization- Inner circle: absence of vascularity.

tibial tendon, because the examination and findings may erroneously mimic a posterior tibial tendon dysfunction. The pain is localized between the navicular and calcaneus, 1 cm proximal to the scaphoid tuberosity and posteriorly in relation to the posterior tibial tendon, being more distal than the usual pain caused by this tendon; there can also be some pain-related difficulty in monopodal support and a slight drop of the medial longitudinal arch of the foot secondary to moving the talus to a vertical position.[10]

At the perimalleolar level, the swelling may be absent or less evident because there is not as much fluid in the synovial sheath as in episodes of synovitis of the posterior tibial tendon rupture. The too-many-toes sign is negative (**Figs. 11** and **12**). In most patients less than 50 years old, the mechanism of injury is secondary to an episode of torsion without relation to a particular sports activity. Injuries in patients more than 50 years old are generally not correlated with prior traumatic pain episodes, which suggests a degenerative cause. In its most frequent presentation, it is associated with various posterior tibial tendon lesions. It is difficult to establish a connection with the lesion grade because we have seen it in grades II and III.

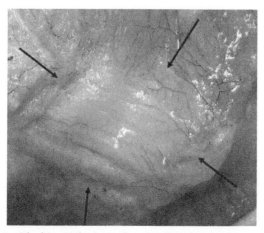

Fig. 8. SM ligament with chines ink. Avascular area between arrows.

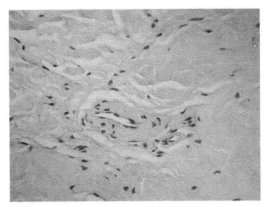

Fig. 9. Histological study SM ligament (central area: absence of vascularity).

COMPLEMENTARY TESTS

In minor lesions or ruptures, radiographic images are normal; however, with higher grade lesions, the head of the talus drops and some investigators have described midfoot abduction without the navicular uncovering the head of the talus (**Fig. 13**A, B). Therefore, the most useful complementary tests are the ultrasonography and noncontrast (ideally microcoil), magnetic resonance imaging (MRI) with axial, coronal, and sagittal cuts of the foot. With a high-resolution ultrasound scanner, the superomedial bundle can be identified and measured, moving the probe from the sustentaculum tali to the navicular. On echographs the superomedial bundle has a fibrillar texture and a smooth concavity that contains the head of the talus.

In the study by Harish and colleagues,[11] it was possible to isolate and identify the posterior tibial tendon and the superomedial bundle at the level of the navicular in 92.5% of the healthy volunteers, whereas it could be identified at the level of the sustentaculum tali in 100% of cases. According to Mengiardi and colleagues,[10] the average size of the bundles is: superomedial bundle, 3.2 mm; inferoplantar bundle, 4.0 mm; oblique bundle, 2.8 mm. Therefore, the superomedial bundle is considered abnormal when it measures 5 mm or more, although other investigators accept up to 4 mm.[10]

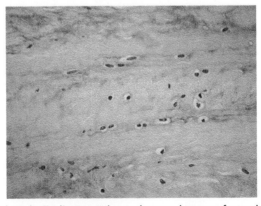

Fig. 10. Histological study SM ligament (central area: absence of vascularity).

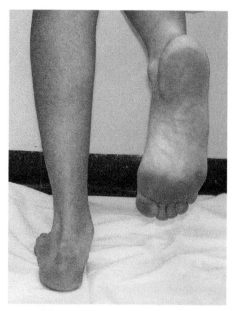

Fig. 11. Difficulty in monopodal support in a patient with superomedial ligament lesion.

The MRI sagittal cuts may show edema in the plantar region of the head of the talus and a thicker superomedial bundle secondary to fibrosis, and even a signal of a torn calcaneonavicular ligament (**Figs. 14** and **15**). The axial cuts of the foot show the infer-oplantar bundle, which is generally not involved and is difficult to explore surgically. The orientation of the ligament fibers makes the diagnosis of the lesion difficult, and its interpretation depends on the cut; we therefore recommend microcoil use in the MRI. Computed tomography scans are not useful for the diagnosis.

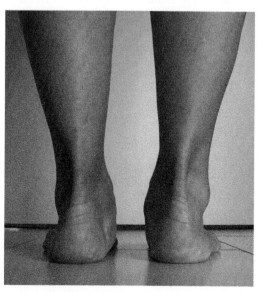

Fig. 12. Too many toe sign negative. Drop of the longitudinal arch (patient with SM lesion).

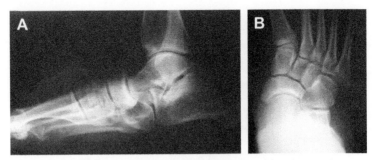

Fig. 13. (*A*) Xr AP view (without abduction). (*B*) Xr lateral view (talus drop).

CLASSIFICATION

Although many classifications have been described,[5] is difficult to make the clinical diagnosis of the degree of the ligament injury or the association with posterior tibial tendon dysfunction. We have found acute and chronic ruptures caused by different mechanisms; trauma prevailed in the acute setting. Chronic injuries may be isolated or associated with some degree of posterior tibial tendon dysfunction. In surgery, we have seen a range of conditions from simple elongations to small and large ruptures, located centrally or around the superomedial bundle (**Figs. 16–18**).

TREATMENT

Once the diagnosis is made, treatment is almost always surgery, because orthopedic treatment has not given good results. Numerous procedures are described in the literature, among them direct suturing of the calcaneonavicular ligament with nonabsorbable material, using the anterior portion of the deltoid ligament, the posterior tibial tendon, or the split anterior tibial tendon for the repair, with excellent results in 77% of cases.[5,12] In in vitro tests, the lateral peroneus longus tendon is used for tendon

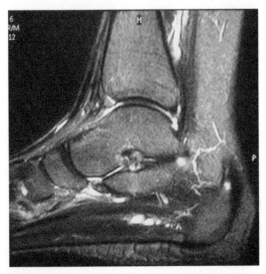

Fig. 14. MRI SM ligament rupture.

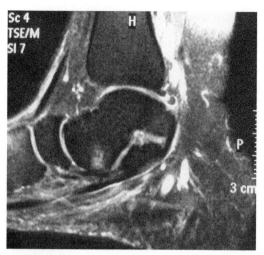

Fig. 15. MRI: talus head edema.

reconstruction.[13] In our experience, most lesions are located in the center of the superomedial ligament, perpendicular to the ligament and of variable length. In single acute ruptures of less than 1 cm, we resect the edges of the lesion, which in most cases is located in the avascular central portion of the superomedial bundle, and subsequently suture the remaining ends with separate resorbable stitches (Vicryl 1) (**Fig. 19**). In ruptures greater than 1 cm that have been developing for more than 4 to 6 months, a Z-tenotomy of the posterior tibial tendon is added to the procedure described earlier, and then the tendon is shortened by 7 mm to protect the superomedial bundle suture (**Fig. 20A–C**).

In calcaneonavicular ligament ruptures associated with posterior tibial tendon dysfunction stage II (in all its forms) ligament repair is performed associated with the treatment of stage II. If the calcaneonavicular ligament rupture is associated with a stage III dysfunction of the posterior tibial tendon, repair is not required whenever a talonavicular arthrodesis is indicated. The postoperative treatment for the simple suture is a nonwalking short plaster cast, forefoot inverted and in forced adduction for 6 weeks, then a rocker-bottom walking brace for 2 to 4 weeks. The preliminary postoperative results are good; patients have returned to their daily activities without pain and with improved internal longitudinal arch height and forefoot abduction.

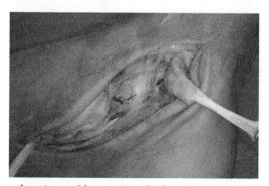

Fig. 16. Rupture less than 1 cm with posterior tibial tendon tenotomy.

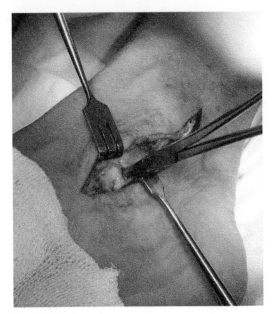

Fig. 17. Rupture of the SM ligament.

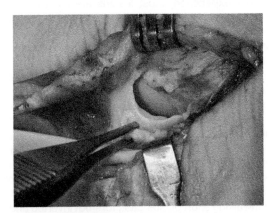

Fig. 18. Complete rupture of the SM ligament.

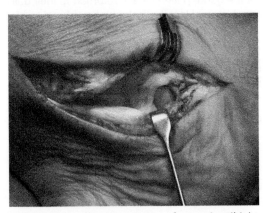

Fig. 19. Minor injury of the SM, withour tenotomy of posterior tibial tendon.

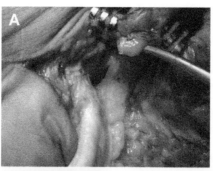

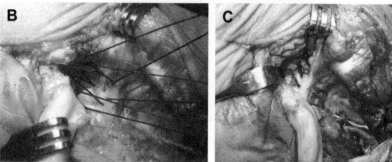

Fig. 20. (*A*) Suture of the SM injury with posterior tibial tendon tenotomy. (*B, C*) SM ligament repairs.

SUMMARY

The calcaneonavicular ligament lesion may be single or related to posterior tibial tendon involvement; the clinical and image-based diagnosis is difficult, without pathognomonic signs. The diagnosis is made during surgery and the calcaneonavicular ligament should always be explored whenever the posterior tibial tendon is involved.

ACKNOWLEDGEMENTS

To Ezequiel Zaindemberg (anatomist) MD and Eduardo Santini Araujo (pathologist) MD, for their excellent academic work.

REFERENCES

1. Taniguchi A, Yasuhito T, Takakura Y, et al. Anatomy of the spring ligament. J Bone Joint Surg Am 2003;85:2174–8.
2. Patil V, Ebraheim N, Frogrameni A, et al. Morphometric dimensions of the calcaneonavicular (spring) ligament. Foot Ankle Int 2007;28(8):927–32.
3. Rule J, Yao L, Seeger LL. Spring ligament of the ankle: normal MR anatomy. Am J Roentgenol 1993;161:1241–4.
4. Deland JT. The adult acquired flatfoot and spring ligament complex: pathology and implications for treatment. Foot Ankle Clin 2001;6:129–35.
5. Gazdag AR, Cracchiolo A 3rd. Rupture of the posterior tibial tendon: evaluation of injury of the spring ligament and clinical assessment of tendon transfer and ligament repair. J Bone Joint Surg Am 1997;79:675–81.

6. Sarrafian SK. Anatomy of the foot and ankle. Philadelphia: JB Lippincott; 1983. p. 157–75.
7. Davis WH, Sobel M, Dicarlo EF, et al. Gross, histological, and microvascular anatomy and biomechanical testing of the spring ligament complex. Foot Ankle Int 1996;17:95–102.
8. Hardy RH. Observations on the structure and properties of the plantar calcaneo-navicular ligament in man. J Anat 1951;85:135–9.
9. Burgos J, Loncharich E, Macklin Vadell A, et al. Vascularización del ligamento calcáneo-escafoideo. Tobillo y Pie/Tornazelo e Pé 2010;2(2):28–33.
10. Mengiardi B, Zanetti M, Schottle P, et al. Spring ligament complex: MR imaging-anatomic correlation and findings in asymptomatic subjects. Radiology 2005; 237(1):242–9.
11. Harish S, Jan E, Finlay K, et al. Sonography of the superomedial part of the spring ligament complex of the foot: a study of cadavers and asymptomatic volunteers. Skeletal Radiol 2007;36:221–8.
12. Deland JT, Annoczky S, Thompson FM. Adult acquired flatfoot deformity at the talonavicular joint: reconstruction of the spring ligament in an in vitro model. Foot Ankle Int 1992;13:327–32.
13. Thorardson DB, Schmotzer H, Chon J. Reconstruction with tenodesis in an adult flatfoot model: a biomechanical evaluation of four methods. J Bone Joint Surg Am 1995;77:1557–64.

Use of Poly(Ether Ether Ketone) Cages in Foot and Ankle Surgery

Daniel Niño Gomez, MD*, Santiago Eslava, MD,
Anain Federico, MD, Yearson Diego, MD, Guillermo Arrondo, MD,
German Joannas, MD*

KEYWORDS

• PEEK cage • PEEK foot fusion • Column-lengthening PEEK • Alternative bone graft

KEY POINTS

• The modulus elasticity of poly(ether ether ketone) (PEEK) is similar to bone.
• There are no donor site problems with PEEK.
• PEEK does not have the drawbacks associated with allografts.
• PEEK cages are radiolucent.
• Wedge-shaped cages are used for column lengthening.
• Box-shaped cages are used for height loss or in cavities.
• Bone fusion rates are high when PEEK cages are filled with autologous bone.
• PEEK is an effective alternative when structural bone graft is needed.

INTRODUCTION

Bone grafting is indicated for many surgical procedures on the foot and ankle, including arthrodesis, repair of complex fractures and malunions, and filling of defects within bones on the foot. When considering bone-grafting alternatives, the surgeon needs material that provides osteogenic cells (which differentiate into cells that are capable of producing bone),[1] osteoinductive factors (which produce elements that induce bone formation), and an osteoconductive matrix (which provides a scaffold that supports bone growth).[1]

Tricortical iliac crest bone graft is accepted to be the best option when structural defects or cavities need to be filled.[2,3] This graft can provide satisfactory clinical results and fusion rates. The complication rates of the donor site are around 20%,[4] some of the most common being pain, nerve damage, cosmetic problems, hemorrhage, hernia, fractures, and ureteral injury.[1] Arrington and colleagues[5]

Instituto Dupuytren, Avenida Belgrano 3460, Capital Federal, Buenos Aires, Argentina
* Corresponding authors.
E-mail addresses: dgomez@intramed.net; germanjoannas@hotmail.com

Foot Ankle Clin N Am 17 (2012) 449–457
http://dx.doi.org/10.1016/j.fcl.2012.07.001
1083-7515/12/$ – see front matter © 2012 Elsevier Inc. All rights reserved.

foot.theclinics.com

identified 2 different groups: minor complications (which respond to aggressive nonoperative intervention such as aspiration and oral antibiotics), including superficial hematomas, superficial seromas, and superficial infections; and major complications (which need either a major change in treatment, prolonged hospitalization, or a return to the operating room), including donor-defect hernias, vascular injuries, nerve injuries, deep infections, deep hematomas, and iliac wing fractures.

Postoperative pain is the most common complication.[1] Fernyhough and colleagues[6] found a 29% incidence of chronic pain at the donor site in their retrospective study. Goulet and colleagues[7] noted in their review that pain was the most common complaint during the first 6 months (38%). This figure dropped to 18% 2 years after surgery. DeOrio and Farber[8] reviewed morbidity after harvest of anterior iliac crest bone graft for procedures involving the foot and ankle. Of their patients, 84% were limited in their activities because of pain at the bone graft site for less than 4 weeks; 7% had pain that resolved by 8 weeks; 4% had pain that resolved within 6 months; and 3% had limiting pain for more than 7 months. Pain can also be a result of a neurologic injury (lateral femoral cutaneous nerve or cluneal nerves). Meralgia paresthetica describes symptoms that are associated with injury of the lateral cutaneous nerve. DeOrio and Farber[8] reported postprocedure numbness in 29% of patients. This numbness resolved in 42%, improved in 29%, and remained unchanged in 29%. It is important that surgeons know the local anatomy of the site from which they take the graft, as this will aid in significantly decreasing the pain related to nerve injury.

Fractures of pelvic iliac wing after anterior iliac crest harvest have been described. Arrington and colleagues[5] described 2 cases in 414 patients. In both cases, harvesting of the anterior iliac crest bone graft was noted to be too close to the anterior superior iliac spine, causing the fracture of the anterior superior iliac spine from the iliac wing. Both patients were treated nonoperatively.

The most dramatic complication, though rare, is herniation of abdominal contents through the donor defect.

The application of allograft bone is another option in foot and ankle surgery. Allografts are advantageous because the quantity of allograft bone available to a given patient is essentially unlimited. The use of allograft bone would eliminate a second incision site (with no cosmetic problems), the operative risk associated with this procedure is low, and there is less pain and morbidity associated with the iliac crest donor site.[9] Allografts have several drawbacks. Such a graft is generally not as effective clinically as a comparable autograft,[10] and there is some risk of transmission of hepatitis B, hepatitis C, and human immunodeficiency virus (HIV).[9,10] Moreover, in Argentina the use of allografts increases the cost of surgery.

Considering this morbidity of the donor site and problems with allografts, the authors have decided to use poly(ether ether ketone) (PEEK) cages to replace iliac crest bone grafting in various procedures. PEEK polymers are obtained by step-growth polymerization by the dialkylation of bisphenolate salts. PEEK is a semicrystalline thermoplastic with excellent mechanical and chemical resistance properties that are retained up to high temperatures.

The Young modulus of PEEK is 3.6 GPa and its tensile strength 90 to 100 MPa. PEEK has a glass transition temperature at around 143°C (289°F) and melts around 343°C (662°F). It is highly resistant to thermal degradation as well as attack by both organic and aqueous environments. It is attacked by halogens and strong Bronsted and Lewis acids, as well as some halogenated compounds and aromatic hydrocarbons at high temperatures (**Fig. 1**).[11]

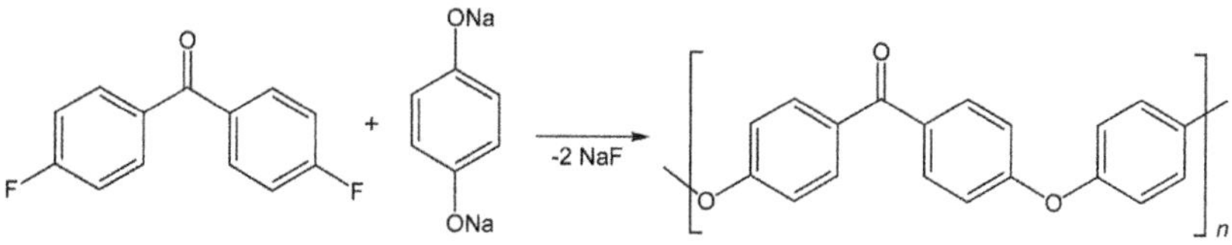

Fig. 1. Qualitative formula of PEEK.

MATERIAL AND METHODS

During 2009 and 2010, 32 cages were used in different procedures in 22 patients (14 females and 8 males) (**Table 1**):

- 3 subtalar joint fusions
- 4 subtalar joint fusions with lateral column lengthening in posterior tibial tendon dysfunction (PTTD)
- 11 lateral column lengthening in PTTD
- 1 calcaneocuboid joint fusion
- 3 first metatarsophalangeal (MTP) joint fusions after failed Keller procedure

All patients were treated at the foot and ankle service in the Instituto Dupuytren. The authors were unable to obtain cages for foot surgery in Argentina; therefore, together with a local company (Equimedica SRL, Buenos Aires), they designed cages for foot and ankle surgery. Two different types of cage were made: box-shaped cages of 20 × 20 mm and 15 × 15 mm, and wedge-shaped cages of 20 × 20 mm and 15 × 15 mm. For both groups, different sizes were made: 7, 9, 11, and 13 (**Fig. 2**).

The entire structure is radiolucent, and both designs have been used. Wedge shapes are indicated for lateral column lengthening and subtalar fusion; and the box shape is used when cavities or height loss is the main concern. PEEK cages were always filled with cancellous bone resected from the fusion site or the calcaneal lateral wall, when medial slide osteotomy and lateral column lengthening was performed.

The wedge-shaped PEEK cage was the most commonly used (28 cases), 15 for lateral column lengthening (8 fixed with titanium staples and 7 with 4.0-mm cannulated screws) and 13 for subtalar joint fusions (all fixed with 2 6.5-mm cannulated screws) (**Figs. 3–6**).[12]

A box shape was used only for failed Keller procedures that needed MTP fusions (3 cases) and length restoration in calcaneocuboid joint fusion (1 case) (**Fig. 7**).

RESULTS

All 22 patients were evaluated with plain radiography and computed tomography (CT) as well as clinically during the follow-up. Radiographically the fusion status was rated as fused, delayed union, or pseudoarthrosis.[13,14]

When there was absence of a solid fusion mass but no evidence of halo around the implant and absence of pain with articular motion, this was classed as delayed union.

Pseudoarthrosis was suspected if there was persistent localized pain, worsened with activity, relieved with rest, and/or hardware failure, and radiographic evidence of pseudoarthrosis (lack of bridging callus, areas of lucency, or lack of a solid fusion mass).[15]

Bone fusion was obtained in 21 patients (14 weeks average); one patient (#21) had a delayed union (20 weeks).

One patient (#15) had a 4-mm cage dorsal migration based on radiographs and CT, but no second procedure was needed because she had no complaints.

Table 1
Patients, hardware, and procedure

Patient #	Hardware	Procedure
1	20 × 20 × 9 mm cage + 22 × 22 mm Ti staple	Calcaneocuboid joint fusion
2	15 × 15 × 11 mm cage + dorsal plate	First MTP joint fusion
3	20 × 20 × 9 mm cage + 6.5 mm CS + 22 × 22 mm Ti staple	Lateral column lengthening in PTTD
4	Two 20 × 20 × 9 mm cages + 2 6.5 × 90 mm CS	Subtalar joint fusion
5	15 × 15 × 11 mm cage + dorsal plate	First MTP joint fusion
6	15 × 15 × 7 mm cage + 2 6.5 mm CS + 4.0 × 30 mm CS	Lateral column lengthening in PTTD
7	Two 20 × 20 × 11 mm cages + 20 × 20 × 7 mm cage + 6.5 mm CS + 25 × 22 mm Ti staple	Subtalar joint fusion with lateral column lengthening in PTTD
8	15 × 15 × 7 mm cage + 10 mm step plate + 4.0 × 30 mm CS	Lateral column lengthening in PTTD
9	20 × 20 × 9 mm cage + 10 mm step plate + 22 × 22 mm Ti staple	Lateral column lengthening in PTTD
10	15 × 15 × 7 mm cage + dorsal plate	First MTP joint fusion
11	20 × 20 × 11 mm cage + 10 mm step plate + 22 × 22 mm Ti staple	Lateral column lengthening in PTTD
12	Two 20 × 20 × 9 mm cages + 15 × 15 × 9 mm cage + 2 6.5 × 85 mm CS + 22 × 22 mm Ti staple	Subtalar joint fusion with lateral column lengthening in PTTD
13	20 × 20 × 11 mm cage + 6.5 × 85 mm CS + 22 × 22 mm Ti staple	Lateral column lengthening in PTTD
14	Two 20 × 20 × 13 mm cages + 2 6.5 × 85 mm CS	Subtalar joint fusion
15	20 × 20 × 11 mm cage + 10 mm step plate + 16 × 15 mm Ti staple	Lateral column lengthening in PTTD
16	20 × 20 × 7 mm cage + 10 mm step plate + 16 × 15 mm Ti staple	Lateral column lengthening in PTTD
17	Two 20 × 20 × 11 mm cages + 15 × 15 × 7 mm cage + 6.5 × 85 mm CS + 4.0 × 30 mm CS	Subtalar joint fusion with lateral column lengthening
18	Two 20 × 20 × 13 mm cages + 15 × 15 × 9 mm cage + 6.5 × 85 mm CS + 4.0 × 34 mm CS	Subtalar joint fusion with lateral column lengthening
19	20 × 20 × 9 mm cage + 10 mm step plate + 4.0 × 28 mm CS	Lateral column lengthening in PTTD
20	20 × 20 × 11 mm cage + 6.5 × 90 mm CS + 4.0 × 30 mm CS	Lateral column lengthening in PTTD
21	15 × 15 × 11 mm cage + 6.5 × 85 mm CS	Subtalar joint fusion
22	20 × 20 × 11 mm cage + 10 mm step plate + 4.0 × 30 mm CS	Lateral column lengthening in PTTD

Abbreviations: CS, cannulated screw; MTP, metatarsophalangeal; PTTD, posterior tibial tendon dysfunction.

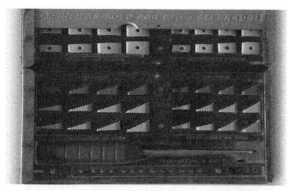

Fig. 2. The two different types of PEEK cage design: box-shaped and wedge-shaped.

A fifth metatarsal stress fracture happened at 6 months postoperatively followed by a fourth metatarsal stress fracture at 9 months in the same patient (#9), probably because of lateral overlengthening, which healed with conservative treatment.

No local complications were reported at the donor site.

DISCUSSION

There are more than 200 publications on the use of the PEEK implant on PubMed, the majority being related to spine surgery. No reports were found on the use of PEEK in foot and ankle surgery.

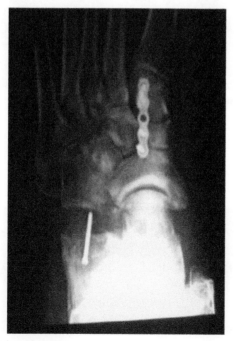

Fig. 3. Lateral column lengthening.

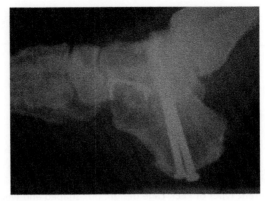

Fig. 4. Subtalar fusion.

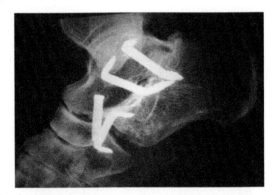

Fig. 5. Tarsal arthrodesis.

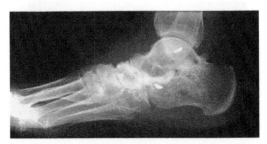

Fig. 6. Two years after surgery.

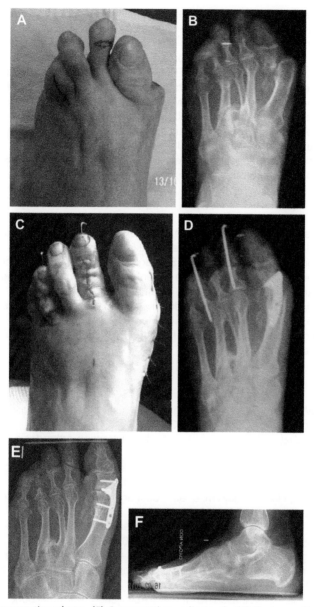

Fig. 7. (*A*) Preoperative photo. (*B*) Preoperative radiograph. (*C*) Postoperative photo. (*D*) Postoperative radiograph. (*E, F*) Postoperative (1 year) radiographs of an akin osteotomy.

The PEEK cage demonstrated absence of cytotoxicity and mutagenicity in an in vitro study.[16] The modulus of elasticity of PEEK is similar to bone. Lee and colleagues[17] showed that patients treated with posterior lumbar interbody fusion (PLIF) using harvested local bone inserted into a PEEK cage had a high rate of fusion: The 6-month fusion rate of the segment was 86.7%, which increased to 90.0% at 12 months (Three-dimensional CT scans were performed to check this). In the authors' study, bone fusion was obtained in 95% of the patients within 14 weeks. Perhaps this difference between series is related to differences in biomechanics.

Implantation of empty PEEK cages after anterior cervical discectomy shows an unexpectedly low rate of fusion according to radiologic criteria (bony fusion was present at 71.7%).[18] In 2008 Liao and colleagues[19] obtained 74% bone fusion after filling the cages with cancellous allograft bone. Allograft bone is not often available in Argentina because it is very expensive. It has some risk of bacterial contamination and viral transmission, albeit very small.[20,21]

Empty cages or cages with cancellous allograft bone were not used by the authors, the rates of fusion being judged to be low.

The use of bone morphogenetic protein for filling the cage has been associated with a greater amount of resorption and migration of the implant.[22]

SUMMARY

PEEK cages are an effective alternative when structural bone graft is needed for different fusions around the foot and ankle.

Bone fusion rates are high when PEEK cages are filled with autologous bone.

No difference in consolidation time in patients was noticed between the cages fixed with staples and those fixed with cannulated screws.

Nerve damage, residual pain at the donor site, and cosmetic problems are avoided with the use of PEEK cages.

There is no risk of transmission of hepatitis B, hepatitis C, and HIV when using PEEK cages.

REFERENCES

1. Boone DW. Complications of iliac graft and bone grafting alternatives in foot and ankle surgery. Foot Ankle Clin 2003;8:1–14.
2. Zion I, Shabat S, Marin L, et al. Subtalar distraction arthrodesis using a ramp cage. Orthopedics 2003;26(11):1117–9.
3. Carr JB, Hansen ST, Benirschke SK. Subtalar distraction bone block fusion for late complications of os calcis fracture. Foot Ankle 1998;9:81–6.
4. Castro FP Jr, Holt RT, Majd M, et al. A cost analysis of two anterior cervical fusion procedures. J Spinal Disord 2000;13:511–4.
5. Arrington ED, Smith W, Chambers HG, et al. Complications of iliac crest bone graft harvesting. Clin Orthop Relat Res 1996;(329):300–9.
6. Fernyhough JC, Schimandle JJ, Weigel MC, et al. Chronic donor site pain complicating bone graft harvesting from the posterior iliac crest for spinal fusion. Spine 1992;17:1474–9.
7. Goulet JA, Senunas LE, DeSilva GL, et al. Autogenous iliac crest bone graft. Complications and functional assessment. Clin Orthop Relat Res 1997;(339):76–81.
8. DeOrio JK, Farber DC. Morbidity associated with anterior iliac crest bone grafting in foot and ankle surgery. Foot Ankle Int 2005;26(2):147–51.
9. Dolan CM, Henning JA, Anderson JG, et al. Randomize prospective study comparing tri-cortical iliac crest autograft to allograft in the lateral column lengthening component for operative correction of adult acquired flatfoot deformity. Foot Ankle Int 2007;28(1):8–12.
10. Catanzariti A, Karlock L. The application of allograft bone in foot and ankle surgery. J Foot Ankle Surg 1995;35(5):440–51.
11. PEEK. Available at: http://en.wikipedia.org/wiki/PEEK. Accessed March 1, 2012.

12. Myerson M. Reconstructive foot and ankle surgery. 1st edition. Elsevier/Saunders; 2005.
13. Sengupta DK, Truumees E, Patel CK, et al. Outcome of local bone versus autogenous iliac crest bone graft in the instrumented posterolateral fusion of the lumbar spine. Spine 2006;31(9):985–91.
14. Blount KJ, Krompinger WJ, Maljanian R, et al. Moving toward a standard for spinal fusion outcomes assessment. J Spinal Disord 2002;15(1):16–23.
15. Dawson EG, Clader TJ, Bassett LW. A comparison of different methods used to diagnose pseudoarthrosis following posterior spinal fusion for scoliosis. J Bone Joint Surg Am 1985;67:1153–9.
16. Katzer A, Marquardt H, Westendorf J, et al. Polyetheretherketone—cytotoxicity and mutagenicity in vitro. Biomaterials 2002;23(8):1749–59.
17. Lee JH, Lee JH, Park JW, et al. Fusion rates of a morselized local bone graft in polyetheretherketone cages in posterior lumbar interbody fusion by quantitative analysis using consecutive three-dimensional computed tomography scans. Spine J 2011;11(7):647–53.
18. Pechlivanis I, Thuring T, Brenke C, et al. Non-fusion rates in anterior cervical discectomy and implantation of empty polyetheretherketone cages. Spine (Phila Pa 1976) 2011;36(1):15–20.
19. Liao JC, Niu CC, Chen WJ, et al. Polyetheretherketone (PEEK) cage filled with cancellous allograft in anterior cervical discectomy and fusion. Int Orthop 2008; 32(5):643–8.
20. Campbell DG, Li P, Oakeshott RD. HIV infection of human cartilage. J Bone Joint Surg Br 1996;78:22–5.
21. Tomford WW, Starkweather RJ, Goldman MH. A study of the clinical incidence of infection in the use of banked allograft bone. J Bone Joint Surg Am 1981;63: 244–8.
22. Vaidya R, Sethi A, Bartol S, et al. Complications in the use of rhBMP-2 in PEEK cages for interbody spinal fusions. J Spinal Disord Tech 2008;21:557–62.

Joint-Preserving Procedure for Moderate Hallux Rigidus

A. Migues, MD[a], Gastón Slullitel, MD[b],*

KEYWORDS

- Hallux rigidus • Joint preservation • Degenerative arthritis • Hallux limitus

KEY POINTS

- Hallux rigidus is a condition characterized by pain and restriction in motion of the first metatarsophalangeal joint, especially in dorsiflexion.[1]
- The ultimate goal of the treatment is to correct the underlying deformity, relieve pain, obtain long-term functional results, and have the shortest period of rehabilitation.
- When pain is present both in maximum dorsiflexion and in mid range of motion, which is the most common scenario, the main choice is to perform a decompressive osteotomy.

INTRODUCTION

Hallux rigidus is a condition characterized by pain and restriction in motion of the first metatarsophalangeal (MTP) joint, especially in dorsiflexion.[1] Symptoms commonly associated with degenerative arthritis of the first MTP joint were initially reported by Davies-Colley[2] in 1887, although Cotterill[3] is credited with proposing the term hallux rigidus. According to the etiology, hallux rigidus can be classified as primary (hallux limitus) or secondary.

Surgical treatment depends on the etiology and severity of the deformity.

Operative procedures are divided into joint-preserving techniques (cheilectomy, phalanx, and first metatarsal osteotomies) and joint-sacrificing techniques (arthrodesis, arthroplasty). The ultimate goal of the treatment is to correct the underlying deformity, relieve pain, obtain long-term functional results, and have the shortest period of rehabilitation.

This article presents a review of the literature and analyzes biomechanical aspects of hallux rigidus, its classification, and etiology, and discusses the available treatment options in the literature along with the authors' preferred approach.

[a] Institute of Orthopaedics "Carlos E. Ottolenghi," Italian Hospital of Buenos Aires, Buenos Aires, Argentina; [b] Institute of Orthopadics "Dr. Jaime Slullitel", Pueyrredon 1027, Rosario, Santa Fe, Argentina
* Corresponding author.
E-mail address: gslullitel@yahoo.com.ar

Foot Ankle Clin N Am 17 (2012) 459–471
http://dx.doi.org/10.1016/j.fcl.2012.06.006
1083-7515/12/$ – see front matter © 2012 Elsevier Inc. All rights reserved.

CLASSIFICATION

In 1988 Hattrup and Johnson[4] published the most common classification system used in the orthopedic literature. It is based on radiographic changes of the first MTP joint on standing anteroposterior and lateral radiographic examination of the foot. Grade I changes consist of mild to moderate osteophyte formation with preservation of joint space. Grade II changes exist if there is less than 50% narrowing of joint space, subchondral sclerosis, and moderate osteophyte formation. Grade III changes result when there is marked osteophyte formation and more than 50% loss of visible joint space, with or without subchondral cyst formation. This classification has prognostic and therapeutic merit, because joint-sparing procedures are used for grade I and II diseases. This treatment protocol is supported by the reported results, which approach 90% good outcomes when a cheilectomy is performed for stages I or II, but success drops down to less than 50% if the same procedure is performed for stage III.

Lately Coughlin and Shurnas[5] have introduced a new classification method, adding a Grade 4 stage, using clinical information to classify the pathology. This classification includes the assessment of pain pattern. According to this, late stages are characterized for pain in the mid range of motion of the 1° MTP joint. There are no joint-sparing procedures for this heterogeneous group of patients. The authors believe that joint decompressive osteotomies may fill this therapeutic gap, and may be considered to preserve the joint motion.

ETIOLOGY

Although various causes have been proposed for hallux rigidus, its exact etiology has yet to be elucidated. Trauma or ostechondritis dissecans may damage the articular surfaces of the MTP joint.[6] Several biomechanical and structural factors may play a role in the development of hallux rigidus. Nilsonne[6] proposed that a long first metatarsal may increase the stress concentrated at the MTP joint during toe-off. Lambrinudi[7] theorized that an elevated first metatarsal leads to excessive plantarflexion of the phalanx and results in a flexion contracture of the joint.

Hypermobility of the first ray, pronation, hallux valgus interphalangeus, hallux valgus, and metatarsus adductus have also been implicated.[8–10] Inflammatory or metabolic conditions such as gout, rheumatoid arthritis, and seronegative arthropathies have also been suggested as possible etiologic factors in hallux rigidus.[11] However, most of these explanations are theoretical and unsupported.

CLINICAL FINDINGS

Hallux rigidus is a condition characterized by pain and restriction of motion of the MTP joint. Patients may have flares of swelling and pain, but over time the flare-ups become more frequent and symptoms become more pronounced.[12] Patients usually refer intolerance to shoe-wear, particularly with high heels.

Physical examination reveals a painful swollen MTP joint with restriction of dorsiflexion. At this point it is particularly important to determine if pain occurs at the mid range of motion or in maximum dorsiflexion. This aspect must be considered to determine the appropriate surgical technique for the patient. Osteophytes around the joint may cause a superficial bursitis, neuritis, or skin ulceration. It is possible to observe an interphalangeal joint hyperextension as compensation of restricted MTP joint dorsiflexion.[13] Pain at the tarso-metatarsal joint may also occur because of this same mechanical compensation.

MANAGEMENT
Nonoperative Treatment

Conservative care is the first indication for patients with hallux rigidus, depending on the extent of arthritis and symptoms. The measures commonly used include foot orthoses, modification in shoe-wear, limitations in activity, physical therapy, and injections with corticosteroid or sodium hyaluronate. There is a lack of high-quality evidence to judge their effectiveness.

Foot orthoses and modified shoe-wear are used to reduced motion and impingement at maximum dorsiflexion.[14] One clinical study found that 47% of patients responded to custom orthoses alone while another 10% responded to simple shoe modifications[15] (Level IV evidence).

Injections with corticosteroid or sodium hyaluronate may provide temporary relief of symptoms. Pons and colleagues[16] prospectively compared the effects of injections with either corticosteroid or sodium hyaluronate. Clinical improvement was observed in both groups at 3 months.

The results of these studies suggest that conservative treatment relieves pain associated with daily activities, and constitute fair evidence (Grade B recommendation).

Operative Management

Surgical correction of hallux rigidus is indicated when conservative treatment fails to relieve pain. At the most basic level, the surgical options involve either preservation or destruction of the articular surfaces, and the decision to pursue one option over the other hinges on the degree of degeneration of articular cartilage.

In cases of severe arthritis, procedures such as arthrodesis, arthroplasty, and joint replacement are indicated. In moderate stages, joint-preserving procedures are preferred. Different techniques have been proposed, but the optimal surgical technique has yet to be defined.

Joint-sparing procedures
Cheilectomy Cheilectomy involves the resection of the dorsal osteophyte and the degenerative portion of the articular surface on the head of the metatarsal.[17] In general, the dorsal one-third of the articular surface is removed. The advantages of a cheilectomy are that it preserves or improves motion, maintains joint stability, has low morbidity, and allows for secondary procedures in the future.[18]

Numerous retrospective case series (Level IV evidence) have reported good results with cheilectomy for early-stage (Grade I and II) hallux rigidus, with success rates ranging from 72% to 100%, and poorer results for advanced disease (Grade III).[19,20] Easley and colleagues[21] reported on their results with cheilectomy in 68 cases of hallux rigidus encompassing all grades of disease at 5-year follow-up (Level IV evidence). There was a 90% satisfaction rate and an average increase in dorsiflexion of the MTP joint from 19° to 39°. Nine feet remained symptomatic, 8 of which had Grade III involvement preoperatively. In all 9, the investigators found pain at the midrange of the arc of motion before surgery, and concluded that this finding indicated advanced arthritis and was a negative prognostic sign. The largest series of cheilectomies to date was published by Coughlin and Shurnas[5] in 2005. In this series, 93 cases were reviewed retrospectively at an average follow-up of 9.6 years (Level IV evidence). Ninety-two percent of the cheilectomies were considered successful, with a mean improvement in dorsiflexion from 15.5° to 38.4°. Nine feet had Grade III changes preoperatively. In 5 of these feet, the procedure failed and was salvaged with an arthrodesis at a mean of 6.9 years. It was concluded that poor results may ensue after cheilectomy in patients with advanced degeneration of the joint.

Complications with this procedure may be observed: osteophyte recurrence, infection, neuroma formation, transient paresthesia, and reflex sympathetic dystrophy.[22]

The authors' perspective on cheilectomy is that the ideal indication is a patient whose complaints are localized to the dorsal exostosis, with minimal or no pain through the midrange of motion. The authors do not consider it a joint-preserving procedure because it removes 30% of the metatarsal head, which may affect the normal biomechanical conditions of the MTP joint. These aspects become important if the patient needs to undergo to a revision arthrodesis.

The consistently favorable results reported in several Level IV studies constitute fair evidence (Grade B recommendation) to support the use of cheilectomy in patients with Grade I and II hallux rigidus. Based on studies with patients with advanced degeneration of the MTP joint, cheilectomy cannot be recommended for Grade III hallux rigidus.

Proximal phalangeal osteotomy Bonney and Macnab[23] first described a dorsal closing wedge osteotomy of the proximal phalanx in 1952 for the treatment of early hallux rigidus in adolescents. Their procedure shifted the limited arc of MTP joint motion dorsally and placed the hallux into more dorsiflexed position, thus allowing for improved function. Moberg[24] published a small series of patients with good outcomes and recommended further investigation of its efficacy. Citron and Neil reviewed 8 patients at an average of 22 years after the procedure (Level IV evidence). While all 8 patients had complete pain relief initially, only 5 were pain free at the latest follow-up. Complications reported included malunion, nonunion, and interphalangeal arthritis.[25]

Several investigators have reported on the use of a dorsal wedge osteotomy in conjunction with a cheilectomy. Blyth and colleagues[8] reviewed a series of 18 patients with a mean follow-up of 4 years. Fourteen patients demonstrated good or excellent results. Thomas and Smith[26] observed a high satisfaction rate, but the average increase in dorsiflexion was only 7°.

Evidence demonstrating the efficacy of Moberg osteotomy, isolated or in combination with cheilectomy, is insufficient (Grade I recommendation) to support its use in the management of hallux rigidus.[27]

Decompressive osteotomy

Biomechanical aspects and rationale of the procedure The proposed causes of a long first metatarsal and metatarsus primus elevatus are the underlying basis for many of the osteotomies designed to treat this disorder. However, the exact role of both conditions as etiologic factors is still controversial.

Coughlin and Shurnas[5] found that a long first metatarsal was no more common in patients with hallux rigidus than in the general population. Besides this aspect, these flat-shaped MTP joints are subjected to an increased axial overload, which may explain its association with hallux rigidus and sesamoid abnormality.

These investigators also demonstrated in a series of 120 patients with hallux rigidus that 94% of the study population had a normal amount of metatarsal elevation. The elevation of the first metatarsal is considered more a consequence than a cause of hallux rigidus, and is more common in its final stages.

The rationale of this osteotomy is to obtain a longitudinal decompression of the joint by means of a proximal translation (shortening) of the metatarsal head, allowing the surrounding soft tissues (plantar fascia, long flexors and extensors, capsule, and so forth) to relax and remodel, initiated by immediate active and passive motion. This rationale is supported by experimental studies suggesting that an increased tension of the plantar fascia causes an abnormal stress on the articular cartilage.[28]

Although not always present, when the first metatarsal head becomes elevated, it prevents the normal dorsal motion of the proximal phalanx on the metatarsal head. In this position, the ground reactive force on the hallux in late stance is altered from a gliding motion to a compression force on the dorsal aspect of the metatarsal head.[29] Consequently, when a metatarsus primus elevatus is present, it has to be restored to its normal position to achieve optimal biomechanical conditions.

In summary, the purpose of this procedure is to decompress the first MTP joint longitudinally, as well as to plantarflex the metatarsal head when it is elevated.

In 2007 the authors started to perform this osteotomy, taking into account its versatility, because it is possible to shorten and/or plantarflex it as desired. Furthermore, it is a simple procedure, very similar to hallux valgus osteotomy, which makes it a reproducible technique. In addition, it is possible to correct an interphalangeal hallux valgus by combining this technique with a similar type of osteotomy.

In 1982, Youngswick[30] described a modification to the Austin (chevron-type) distal osteotomy. His modification consists in making a second osteotomy parallel to the dorsal limb of the V-shaped osteotomy. The purpose of this modification is to translate the metatarsal head plantarward and to decompress the joint. Although he did not report outcomes, he observed complications including fracture, delayed union, and excessive metatarsal shortening.

Oloff and Jhala-Patel[31] reviewed a series of 23 patients (28 feet) who underwent a Youngswick osteotomy for late-stage hallux rigidus. The mean duration of follow-up was 5.7 years. Eighty-five percent of patients reported that they were pleased with their outcome, with 75% of those patients reporting more than 90% improvement in their symptoms.

One of the most popular procedures for moderate cases is the Moberg osteotomy. Kilmartin[32] performed a prospective study comparing phalangeal osteotomy (Moberg) with distal first metatarsal osteotomy. Forty-nine patients underwent phalangeal osteotomy and 59 underwent 3 different metatarsal osteotomies. In the phalangeal group, 65% of the patients were completely satisfied, 24% were satisfied with reservations, and 11% were dissatisfied. There was no difference in dorsiflexion postoperatively. In the first metatarsal osteotomy group, 54% of patients were completely satisfied, 14% satisfied with reservations, and 32% were dissatisfied. Thirty-one percent developed transfer metatarsalgia. This group is a mixture of 3 different osteotomies, so it does not reflect the outcomes achieved with the Youngswick osteotomy.

One of the advantages of this osteotomy is its stability, particularly compared with the distal oblique osteotomy[33]; this is supported by its geometry and the rigid internal fixation. Consequently it is possible to allow the patients to undergo an early range-of-motion protocol, thus preventing the formation of arthrofibrosis, a potential cause of stiffness of the MTP joint.

The authors started to use this technique in index plus forefeet, with good results, which offered the perspective that the decompression alleviates the symptoms, even in those cases with "too much" shortening. It was thus considered that the main cause of the first-ray insufficiency in hallux rigidus is pain, regardless of the metatarsal length. Subsequently the procedure was also performed in index plus-minus (**Fig. 1**) and index minus forefeet (**Fig. 2**), with similar results. At present, the authors indicate this osteotomy without taking care of the metatarsal index. Related to this, there is a lack of metatarsal index analysis in all of the series published in the literature. Some investigators think that this osteotomy is efficient because the shortening can be compensated with plantarflexion.

Another issue to consider is the pattern of pain (dorsal or midrange of motion, or a mixture). Pain is an important characteristic to individualize in the "heterogeneous"

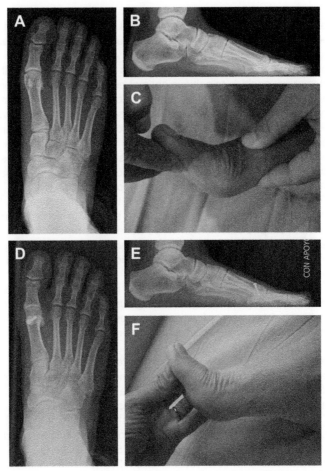

Fig. 1. A 32-year-old woman with a plus-minus forefoot who underwent a decompressive osteotomy. Preoperative radiographs (*A, B*) and clinical dorsiflexion (*C*). Postoperative radiographs (*D, E*) and improvement in clinical dorsiflexion (*F*).

Grade II patients. With the decompressive osteotomy, indications can also be expanded to patients with midrange of motion pain. As such, this is as an advantage over cheilectomy, which is only indicated for isolated maximum dorsiflexion pain.

Some complications did arise. We have had complications, as in one patient who developed an asymptomatic medial deviation of the second toe. This complication has been previously reported. Another patient complained about transfer metatarsalgia and had to undergo a Weil osteotomy of the second metatarsal. Limitations included the lack of long-term follow-up, the small number of patients, and the absence of a control group.

SURGICAL TECHNIQUE

Surgery is performed under local block anesthesia. A tourniquet is applied at the ankle level. The MTP joint is approached through a medial incision. The dorsal and lateral osteophytes are removed. The sesamoid bones are released from the metatarsal head. The great toe is then manipulated until maximal dorsiflexion can be achieved.

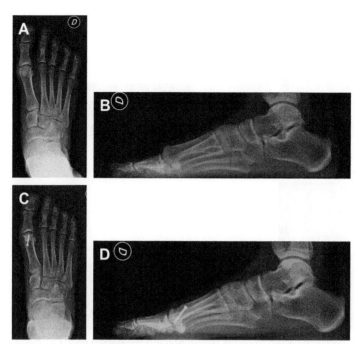

Fig. 2. A 26-year-old woman with a minus forefoot, who underwent a decompressive metatarsal osteotomy. Preoperative (*A, B*) and postoperative (*C, D*) radiographs show how the elevation of the first metatarsal improved postoperatively.

The medial eminence of the head is removed. The integrity of the articular surfaces is examined to assess the chondral lesion pattern (dorsal, central) and for drilling if necessary. Then a chevron-shaped osteotomy is made. The orientation of the plantar arm is performed depending on the amount of plantarflexion desired (**Fig. 3**). A 3-mm slice of bone is cut in the dorsal arm and removed to achieve plantar and proximal displacement of the head combined with medial or later displacement, as needed, to correct the deformity. Fixation is achieved with a 3.0-mm HCS cannulated screw (Synthes, Paoli, PA). In cases with interphalangeal hallux valgus the authors perform an akin osteotomy that is fixed with another 3.0-mm screw, to allow early range of motion (**Fig. 4**). Patients are allowed to bear weight on the operated foot to tolerance with a stiff-bottomed postoperative shoe, and self-directed home physical therapy is started at the first dressing change with passive dorsiflexion-plantarflexion exercises of the first MTP joint.

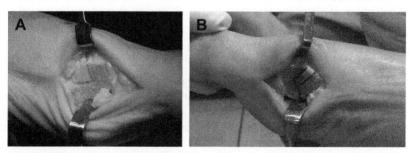

Fig. 3. Two different types of osteotomies. (*A*) reflects a more longitudinal decompression, whereas (*B*) reflects a more plantar flexion osteotomy.

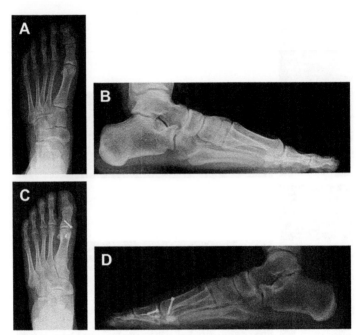

Fig. 4. (*A–D*) A combination of hallux rigidus and interphalangal hallux valgus. Both deformities were addressed.

RESULTS

Between January 2007 and December 2010 the authors performed this osteotomy in 21 patients. There were 14 women and 7 men. The average age was 44.09 years (range 27–61). The follow-up was 21.66 months (range 8–48).

The metatarsal index was as follows: 5 index plus, 6 index plus-minus, and 10 index minus.

The preoperative American Orthopaedic Foot and Ankle Society (AOFAS) score was 39 (range 23–50) and the postoperative score was 81.8 (range 68–92). The average preoperative range of motion of the first MTP joint was 21 degrees (range 11–35), and postoperatively was 29 degrees (range 13–43).

Ninety-one percent of the patients were satisfied with the procedure and stated that they would undergo it again in similar circumstances.

Two complications were observed: one transfer metatarsalgia that underwent a Weil osteotomy in the second metatarsal (**Fig. 5**), and an asymptomatic medial deviation of the second toe (**Fig. 6**).

Joint-Sacrificing Procedures

Keller resection arthroplasty

In 1904, Keller described a technique that resects the base of the proximal phalanx for treatment of hallux valgus with osteoarthritis of the first MTP joint. It was associated with complications such as cock-up deformity, complaints of weakness, and transfer metatarsalgia.[34] However, it is a simple procedure that is still recommended for low-demand and elderly patients.

In 1990, O'Doherty and colleagues[35] published a prospective randomized trial comparing a Keller procedure and arthrodesis of the MTP joint for the diagnosis of

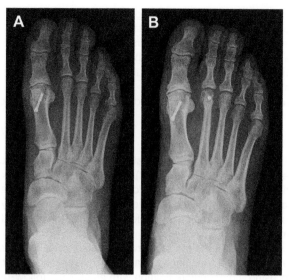

Fig. 5. (*A, B*) A woman who developed a transfer metatarsalgia underwent a Weil osteotomy of the second metatarsal.

hallux valgus and hallux rigidus with a minimum follow-up of 2 years (Level II evidence). The study enrolled 110 patients with an average age of 60.5 years, and reported a satisfactory or excellent result in 98% in the Keller group compared with 95% in the arthrodesis group.

In 2010, Mackey and colleagues[36] also compared the Keller procedure with arthrodesis and concluded that the former is a motion-sparing procedure with equivalent outcomes to those of arthrodesis. Moreover, they observed that it is associated with a more normal pattern of plantar pressure during walking (Level III evidence).

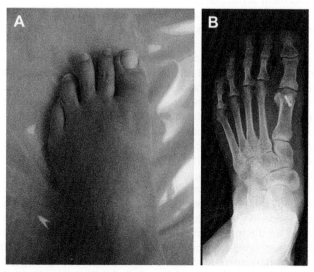

Fig. 6. (*A, B*) Asymptomatic medial deviation of the second toe.

The literature reveals that the Keller procedure is an alternative for advanced (Grade III) hallux rigidus in those patients who reject the arthrodesis. However, its association with cock-up deformity and transfer metatarsalgia is noteworthy.

The favorable results from Level II, III, and IV studies reflect that there is fair evidence (Grade B recommendation) to support the use of resection arthroplasty in older and low-demand patients.

The authors agree with this approach, and seldom indicate this procedure for very low-demand patients.

Arthrodesis

Arthrodesis of the first MTP joint is the mainstay of surgical treatment for patients with advanced stages of hallux rigidus (Grade III). It is particularly indicated in young and more active patients and as an end-stage procedure in recurrent cases. Improvement in joint pain is achieved by eliminating range of motion. However, it may be associated with complications such as malunion, nonunion, arthritis of the interphalangeal joint, or transfer metatarsalgia.[37]

The outcomes reported in the literature reflect fusion rates of between 90% and 100% with different surgical techniques. Flavin and Stephens[38] reported a series of MTP arthrodesis using a dorsal plate fixation with an average follow-up of 18 months (Level IV evidence), which included hallux valgus, hallux rigidus, and nonunion of previous fusions. Radiographic signs of union were observed in all patients at 6 weeks, with significant improvement in clinical outcomes. Goucher and Coughlin[37] published a prospective series of 50 patients who underwent first MTP joint arthrodesis using dome-shaped reamers to prepare the joint and a dorsal plate with a single compression screw. The investigators reported a satisfaction rate of 96% and union rate of 92%, and a significant increase in AOFAS scores at an average follow-up of 16 months. The revision rate was 4% (Level IV evidence).

The series reported in the literature were Level II and IV studies that showed favorable outcomes, and constitute fair evidence (Grade B recommendation) to support the use of arthrodesis for the treatment of advanced-stage hallux rigidus.

Prosthetic replacement arthroplasty

The rationale of using a prosthetic replacement is not only to provide pain relief but also to restore joint motion, which can theoretically be achieved with total metallic implants or hemiarthroplasty.

Gibson and Thomson[39] published a prospective, randomized controlled trial comparing arthrodesis versus total arthroplasty for patients with symptomatic hallux rigidus (Level II evidence). Sixty-three patients were included in the study, with an average age of 55 years. The arthrodesis was performed with flat cuts, and fixed with a cerclage wire and a single Kirschner wire. All of the arthrodeses united. Six of the 39 arthroplasties failed because of loosening of the phalangeal components. The postoperative visual analog scale (VAS) pain scores were significantly reduced in both groups when compared with the preoperative scores. At 2 years after surgery, 40% of patients in the arthroplasty group would not undergo surgery again, compared with only 3% of patients in the arthrodesis group. The conclusion was that the outcomes with the arthrodesis were better than those with the arthroplasty. The poor results published in the literature state that total prosthetic replacement cannot be recommended for the management of hallux rigidus (Grade B recommendation).

The largest review of hemiarthroplasties was performed by Townley and Taranow,[40] which included 279 patients treated with a metallic hemiarthroplasty of the proximal phalanx with follow-up ranging from 8 months to 33 years (Level IV evidence).

Preoperative diagnosis included hallux rigidus, rheumatoid arthritis, and hallux valgus associated with osteoarthritis. Good or excellent results were reported in 95% of patients. There were 9 failures, with only 1 case of clinical and radiographic evidence of loosening. Raikin and colleagues[41] retrospectively compared patients with severe hallux rigidus who were treated with either a metallic hemiarthroplasty or an arthrodesis (Level II evidence). Twenty-one hemiarthroplasties with a mean follow-up of 79 months were compared with 27 arthrodeses with a mean follow-up of 30 months. All arthrodeses united, and 5 of 21 hemiarthroplasties failed. Eight hemiarthroplasties had cut out of the stem through the plantar cortex of the phalanx. The investigators reported that the arthrodesis group had higher satisfaction rates, higher AOFAS scores, and lower VAS pain scores compared with the hemiarthroplasty group. Except for the study by Townley and Taranow, the use of hemiarthroplasty for the treatment of hallux rigidus is supported by conflicting or poor-quality evidence (Grade C recommendation).

Considering the available evidence, the authors do not include MTP joint replacement among the surgical options to treat hallux rigidus.

SUMMARY

Hallux rigidus is a complex disorder, and numerous surgical procedures have been described for its management. Although the optimal technique has yet to be defined, it is important to individualize the degree of arthritis as well as other clinical features (metatarsal index, pain characteristics, and so forth) of each patient to achieve optimal results.

The authors firmly believe that for patients with only dorsal pain, a cheilectomy is the ideal choice because good and reliable results can be achieved. When pain is also present around the joint or is combined, which is the most common scenario, their main choice now is to perform a decompressive osteotomy. The biomechanics of the joint are more adequately restored, soft tissues are relaxed, and remodeling of the contracted tissues is allowed. More investigation has still to be performed to elucidate the origin of this abnormality.

REFERENCES

1. Shereff MD, Baumhauer JF. Hallux rigidus and osteoarthrosis of the first metatarsophalangeal joint. J Bone Joint Surg 1998;80:898–908.
2. Davies-Colley M. Contraction of the metatarsophalangeal joint of the great toe. BMJ 1887;1:728.
3. Cotterill JM. Stiffness of the great toe in adolescents. Br Med J 1888;1:158.
4. Hattrup SJ, Johnson KA. Subjective results of hallux rigidus following treatment with cheilectomy. Clin Orthop Relat Res 1988;226:182–91.
5. Coughlin MJ, Shurnas PS. Hallux rigidus: grading and long term results of operative treatment. J Bone Joint Surg Am 2003;85:2072–88.
6. Nilsonne H. Hallux rigidus and its treatment. Acta Orthop Scand 1930;1:295–303.
7. Lambrinudi P. Metatarsus primus elevatus. Proc R Soc Med 1938;31:1273.
8. Blyth MJ, Mackay DC, Kinninmonth AW. Dorsal wedge osteotomy in the treatment of hallux rigidus. J Foot Ankle Surg 1998;37(1):8–10.
9. Dickerson JB, Green R, Green DR. Long term follow-up of the Green-Waterman osteotomy for hallux limitus. J Am Podiatr Med Assoc 2002;92(10):543–54.
10. Rahman H, Fagg PS. Silicone granulomatous reaction after first metatarsophalangeal hemiarthroplasty. J Bone Joint Surg 1993;75(4):637–9.
11. Kilmartin TE, Wallace WA, Hill TW. Orthotic effect on metatarsophalangeal joint extension. A preliminary study. J Am Podiatr Med Assoc 1991;81(8):414–7.

12. Shurnas PS. Hallux rigidus: etiology, biomechanics and nonoperative treatment. Foot Ankle Clin 2009;14(1):1–8.
13. Feldman RS, Hutter J, Lapow L, et al. Cheilectomy and hallux rigidus. J Foot Surg 1983;22:170–4.
14. Smith RW, Katchis SD, Ayson LC. Outcomes in hallux rigidus patients treated nonoperatively: a long-term follow-up study. Foot Ankle Int 2000;21(11):906–13.
15. Horton GA, Parks YW, Myerson MS. Role of metatarsus primus elevatus in the pathogenesis of hallux rigidus. Foot Ankle Int 1999;20(12):777–80.
16. Pons M, Alvarez F, Solana J, et al. Sodium hyaluronate in the treatment of hallux rigidus. A single-blind, randomized study. Foot Ankle Int 2007;28(1):38–42.
17. Feltham GT, Hanks SE, Markus RE. Age-based outcomes of cheilectomy for the treatment of hallux rigidus. Foot Ankle Int 2001;22(3):192–7.
18. Mulier T, Steenwerckx A, Thienpont E, et al. Results after cheilectomy in athletes with hallux rigidus. Foot Ankle Int 1999;20(4):232–7.
19. Harrison MH, Harvey FJ. Arthrodesis of the first metatarsophalangeal joint for hallux valgus and rigidus. J Bone Joint Surg 1963;45:471–80.
20. McMaster MJ. The pathogenesis of hallux rigidus. J Bone Joint Surg 1978;60(1): 82–7.
21. Easley ME, Davis WH, Anderson RB. Intermediate to long-term follow up of medial-approach dorsal cheilectomy for hallux rigidus. Foot Ankle Int 1999; 20(3):147–52.
22. Fitzgerald JA. A review of long-term results of arthrodesis of the first metatarsophalangeal joint. J Bone Joint Surg 1969;51(3):488–93.
23. Bonney G, Macnab I. Hallux rigidus in the adolescent. J Bone Joint Surg 1952; 34(3):366–85.
24. Moberg E. A simple operation for hallux rigidus. Clin Orthop 1979;142:55–6.
25. Citron N, Neil M. Dorsal wedge osteotomy of the proximal phalanx for hallux rigidus. Long term results. J Bone Joint Surg Br 1987;69(5):835–7.
26. Thomas PJ, Smith RW. Proximal phalanx osteotomy for the surgical treatment of hallux rigidus. Foot Ankle Int 1999;20(1):3–12.
27. Seibert NR, Kadakia AR. Surgical management of hallux rigidus: cheilectomy and osteotomy (phalanx and metatarsal). Foot Ankle Clin 2009;14:9–22.
28. Flavin R, Halpin T, O'Sullivan R, et al. A finite-element analysis study of the metatarsophalangeal joint of the hallux rigidus. J Bone Joint Surg (Br) 2008;90(No. 10): 1334–40.
29. Derner R, Goss K, Postowski HN, et al. A plantarflexory-shortening osteotomy for hallux rigidus: a retrospective analysis. J Foot Ankle Surg 2005;44(5):377–89.
30. Youngswick FD. Modifications of the Austin bunionectomy for treatment of metatarsus primus elevatus associated with hallux limitus. J Foot Surg 1982;21:114–6.
31. Oloff LM, Jhala-Patel G. A retrospective analysis of joint salvage procedures for grades III and IV hallux rigidus. J Foot Ankle Surg 2008;47(3):230–6.
32. Kilmartin TE. Phalangeal osteotomy versus first metatarsal decompression osteotomy for the surgical treatment of hallux rigidus: a prospective study of age-matched and condition-matched patients. J Foot Ankle Surg 2005;44(1):2–12.
33. Malerba F, Milani R, Sartorelli E, et al. Distal oblique metatarsal osteotomy in grade III hallux rigidus: a long term follow-up. Foot Ankle Int 2008;29(7):677–82.
34. Mann RA, Clanton TO. Hallux rigidus: treatment by cheilectomy. J Bone Joint Surg 1988;70(3):400–6.
35. O'Doherty DP, Lowrie IG, Magnussen PA, et al. The management of the painful first metatarsophalangeal joint in the older patient. J Bone Joint Surg 1990; 72(5):839–42.

36. Mackey RB, Thomson AB, Kwon O, et al. The modified oblique Keller capsular interpositional arthroplasty for hallux rigidus. J Bone Joint Surg Am 2010; 92(10):1938–46.
37. Goucher NR, Coughlin MJ. Hallux metatarsophalangeal joint arthrodesis using domed-shaped reamers and dorsal plate fixation: a prospective study. Foot Ankle Int 2006;27(11):869–76.
38. Flavin R, Stephens MM. Arthrodesis of the first metatarsophalangeal joint using a dorsal titanium contoured plate. Foot Ankle Int 2004;25(11):783–7.
39. Gibson A, Thomson CE. Arthrodesis or total replacement arthroplasty for hallux rigidus. Foot Ankle Int 2005;26(9):680–90.
40. Townley TO, Taranow WS. A metallic hemiarthroplasty resurfacing prosthesis for the hallux metatarsophalangeal joint. Foot Ankle Int 1994;15(11):575–80.
41. Raikin SM, Ahmad J, Pour AE, et al. Comparison of arthrodesis and metallic hemi-arthroplasty of the hallux metatarsophalangeal joint. J Bone Joint Surg 2007;89: 1979–85.

Lesser Toes Proximal Interphalangeal Joint Fusion in Rigid Claw Toes

C. Sergio Fernández, MD[a,*], Emilio Wagner, MD[b],
Cristian Ortiz, MD[b]

KEYWORDS

• Rigid claw toes • Proximal interphalangeal joint • Lesser toe • Deformities • PIPJ

KEY POINTS

• Nonsurgical treatments should always be explored before considering surgical intervention.
• In most cases, hallux valgus deformity must be corrected to prevent recurrence of toe deformity.
• Arthrodesis of the lesser toes is the most common procedure to correct the proximal interphalangeal joint deformity.

INTRODUCTION

Lesser toe deformities are a common complaint (more than 20% of office requests)[1] and should not be considered a minor problem because pain and deformity can have a significant impact on the patient's quality of life.

Moreover, a common language and common definitions of every deformity are lacking,[2] and this misunderstanding precludes comparable results among different publications. For the purposes of this discussion, hammertoes are defined as flexion of the proximal interphalangeal joint (PIPJ) with or without interphalangeal joint deformity.[3]

NONSURGICAL TREATMENT

Nonsurgical treatment is the first approach for most patients. It should include a recommendation to wear shoes with wide toe boxes and avoid high heels. Some devices are available off the shelf, including padding for painful calluses, silicone gel pads, and different kinds of strapping devices. Periodic trimming is also helpful, but none of these options produces a permanent correction. If the patient is not satisfied with nonsurgical treatment, surgical options can be recommended.

[a] Foot & Ankle, Clinica Santa Maria, La Gioconda 4344 Dpto 201, Las Condes, Santiago 6761703, Chile; [b] Clinica Alemana, Universidad del Desarrollo, Las Condes, Vitacura 5951, Santiago, Chile
* Corresponding author.
E-mail address: fernandez.sc@gmail.com

Foot Ankle Clin N Am 17 (2012) 473–480
http://dx.doi.org/10.1016/j.fcl.2012.07.004
1083-7515/12/$ – see front matter © 2012 Elsevier Inc. All rights reserved.

SURGICAL TREATMENT

Before specifically addressing the PIPJ deformity, the whole foot must be taken into consideration. Because some forefoot deformities can be related to hindfoot problems (hindfoot-driven forefoot deformity), in some specific cases, flat foot correction or other deformities should be addressed. In most cases, hallux valgus deformity must be corrected to prevent recurrence of toe deformity.

The last consideration before correcting the PIPJ deformity is to evaluate metatarsophalangeal (MTP) deformity or instability. Although it is not the focus of this discussion, MTP dorsiflexion or instability must be corrected with soft tissue lengthening (extensor tendon, dorsal capsule) and sometimes metatarsal shortening with some kind of Weil osteotomy modification.

Although flexible deformities of the PIPJ can be corrected with a flexor to extensor tendon transfer (Girdlestone Taylor procedure), the satisfaction rate varies from 51% to 91% because of generalized stiffness and loss of motion control.[4] On our own patients, the main complaint after small toe deformity correction has been the loss of correction, with minor concern regarding loss of flexibility. Our experience has indicated that our patients prefer a stiff but straight small toe. With this subjective opinion in mind, we are more inclined now to perform procedures on flexible, semiflexible, and rigid PIPJ deformities, which can deliver a straight toe reliably over time, not taking into consideration the remanent motion of the PIPJ. Soft tissue arthroplasties, temporal PIPJ fixation with resorbable pins, or PIPJ fusions have been our choice in recent years, with good results.

Regarding fusion of the PIPJ, the first surgical treatment was described on 1910 by Soule[5] and used a plantar approach and cast. Jones in 1917 first used a dorsal approach, and Higgs and Young[6] analyzed how to improve the stability of the fusion site. Kirschner (K) wire was first described in 1940 by Taylor. Since Du Vries'[7] description in 1956, several modifications to his technique and new proposals to solve this problem have arisen. Simple and complex surgical techniques and different kinds and models of stabilization devices have been used to fuse the PIPJ. Osteosynthesis and fusion site compression have changed the way of obtaining stable and well-positioned fused PIPJs. The way of resecting the articular surfaces is also important. The larger the surface, the better the fusion rate. V-shaped cuts in the proximal phalangeal (F1) condyles and homonymous resection in the middle phalangeal (F2) base present the larger fusion surface and also supply intrinsic stability.[8–11] An adequate coronal angle of the resection avoids toe malrotation. Techniques like peg in the hole are technically demanding and require special hardware.[11–13]

Consideration has to be given to the complete foot, and complete preoperative planning is necessary when dealing with deformities of the toes to achieve best results.[14]

Unpleasant results are not infrequent,[5] and several foot and ankle surgeons believe that conditions of the toe are the least easy to treat and that patients return repeatedly because they are not satisfied with the results. Revision rates vary from 17.8% to 23.7%, and swelling, malrotation, nonunion, and infection are frequently reported.[5] Overall, arthrodesis of the lesser toes is the most common procedure for correcting PIPJ deformity, although similar results have been obtained with stable resection arthroplasty, as reported by Coughlin and colleagues.[10]

The most common fusion techniques used for a PIPJ deformity are:

1. K wire/resorbable pin[9,10,15–18]
2. Interfragmentary compression with screws[19,20]
3. Special devices created specifically for this purpose[21]

K Wire

After articular surface resection, a K wire/resorbable pin is driven through F2 and the distal phalanx (F3) to the tip of the toe. After reduction of the PIPJ, the K wire is reversed toward F1. Attention has to be focused on compressing the fusion site and avoiding spaces between F1 and F2. The K wire is then cut, close to the tip of the toe, and bent or cap covered. The K wire should be removed in a simple office procedure at 3 to 6 weeks. This is a reliable technique that consistently gives a high level of satisfactory results.[10]

The K wire can also be left buried inside F1 and F2, avoiding infection risk and discomfort during extraction of the K wire.[9,15] Resorbable pins have some advantages[22] and obtain the same results as conventional K wires. Resorbable pins are cut just over the skin of the tip of the toe and pushed toward F3 with a special pusher.

Rotational control is also essential in this stabilization and is clinically controlled. Extraction discomfort and infection risk are avoided with this device,[17] but costs have to be considered.

Interfragmentary Compression Screw

Interfragmentary compression screws are available in 2.0, 2.4, and 2.7 mm, and cannulated 2.0 and 3.0 screws can also be used. From proximal to distal, a sliding/gliding hole is drilled, and the selected screw is retrograde-driven from the tip of the toe until its tip appears in the F2 resected base surface. From distal to proximal, the selected drill bit is used to insinuate the F1 medullary canal drill and the screw is driven and tightened, keeping the fusion area under pressure and rotational control.

The technique has few modifications when a cannulated screw is used instead of a solid one. Cannulated screws can be easily inserted and also the guide wire can be used as supplementary stabilization or to stabilize the MTP joint.

Screws of 2.7 mm have a big head that could cause problems related to the nail and the nail bed, with exposure of the screw and infection risk. Screws of 2.0 mm have a limited mechanical resistance and are prone to fracture under normal weight-bearing forces. Screws of 2.4 mm apparently fulfill the ideal characteristics, with a small screw head and sufficient mechanical resistance to support sustained weight bearing, even if fusion has not been achieved.

A special screw has been created for this purpose (Michael Vitek, personal communication, 2010) and is designed to be used antegrade, from the proximal to the intermediate phalanx, achieving interfragmentary compression and avoiding distal interphalangeal joint (DIPJ). This technique keeps the PIPJ in 20 to 25° of flexion.

Special Fixation Devices

Several recently designed devices are available in the orthopedic market. These new devices claim to be simple, safe, and compressive and to achieve early fusion and a low complication rate. These implants are designed specifically to achieve PIPJ fusion. Smart Toe (Memometal Technologies, Rue Baise Pascal, Bruz France), like an endomedullar staple, is claimed to be self-compressive to achieve fusion. Pro-Toe EndoSorb is built with poly(lactic-co-glycolic acid), comes in 1 size, and is said to be simple and easy to use, with cost-effective advantages. The Pro-Toe VO (Wright Medical Technology, Arlington, TN, USA) stainless steel implant comes in 0° and 10° flexion and 1 size. There are some reports with small series of hammertoes treated with these implants with good results, and they have been reported to be "a viable alternative for the treatment of hammertoe." They are also considered useful in diabetic patients because of their specific stability and 98% fusion rate.

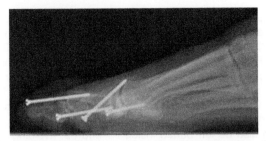

Fig. 1. Lateral radiograph of forefoot area. Note the distal migration of the screw in relation to the second toe. Also note the fracture of the proximal phalanx of the fourth toe.

AUTHORS' PREFERRED APPROACH

Our personal experience with screws begun with 2.7 screws. After a short period during which nail bed disruption and exposure of the screw head occurred in 4 of 10 toes (**Fig. 1**), a decision to use 2.0 screws was made. Fracture of 2 screws in the early postoperative period (**Fig. 2**) led us to decide to use 2.4 screws. Our surgical technique includes a longitudinal approach over the involved joint (**Fig. 3**). We transversely cut the extensor tendon apparatus, resect the collateral ligaments, and then expose the joint. Cartilage is resected from the base of the middle phalanx and the head of the proximal phalanx is resected as much as necessary to obtain a straight toe (**Fig. 4**). In drilling of F2 and F3, retrograde from the distal aspect of the toe proximally, care is taken to place the drill plantar to the F3 distal nail expansion, avoiding nail bed damage or dorsal protrusion of the screw head. The DIPJ is held in mild extension, which has not been a subject of complaint in the postoperative evolution of the patients. The joint is then fixed, preferably with a 2.4-mm screw, maintaining manual compression of the joint (**Fig. 5**). The skin is closed and regular dressings are applied over the involved toes.

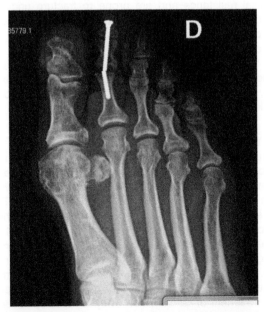

Fig. 2. Anteroposterior view of a foot, in which fracture of the screw is noticed.

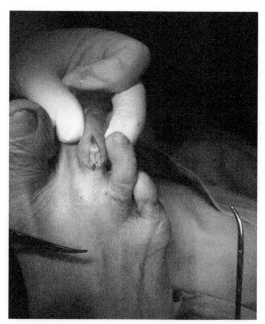

Fig. 3. Intraoperative picture of PIPJ arthrodesis. A longitudinal incision is performed over the PIPJ. Division of extensor tendon and collateral ligaments is performed to access the joint.

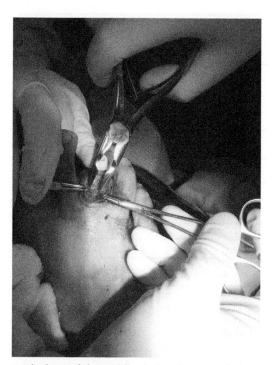

Fig. 4. The cartilage at the base of the middle phalanx is resected. The head of the proximal phalanx is resected as needed to obtain a straight toe with a reduced PIPJ.

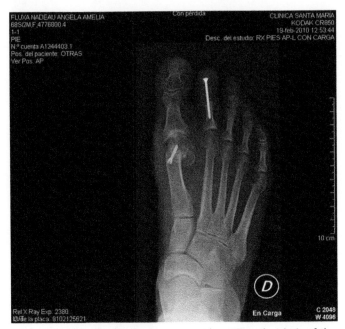

Fig. 5. Final postoperative radiograph of patient with a PIPJ arthrodesis of the second toe. Complete alignment of the toe is achieved.

Table 1
Follow-up

Screw Size	Number	Follow-Up (mo)
2.7	14	12 (6–24)
2.0	25	12 (6–22)
2.4	95	10 (6–20)
Total	134	10,5 (6–24)

Table 2
Mechanical complications with screws

Complication	Screw	Number/Total Screws
Nail bed protrusion	2.7	4/14
Broken screw	2.0	2/12
Dorsal Cortical F1 Fracture	2.4, 2.7	4/109 (95 + 14)

Table 3
Complications in 95 cases with 2.4 screws

Complication	Number/Total
Broken screw	1/95
Nail bed protrusion	0/95
Malposition	3/95

Table 4
Clinical results: patient's satisfaction at 10.5 months

Satisfaction	All Toes		2.4 Toes	
	N°	%	N°	%
Without Complaint	92	69%	70	74%
Minimal Complaint	24	18%	16	17%
Major Complaint	8	6%	5	5%
Dissatisfied	10	7%	4	4%
Total	134	100%	95	100%

RESULTS

We have performed more than 200 PIPJ fusions with screws, most of them with 2.4 screws. So far, 134 procedures have had a minimum of 6 months of follow-up (**Table 1**). Multiple, different but infrequent complications were present in these 134 toes (**Table 2**). Over the last 18 months, all the screws have been 2.4 mm and nevertheless there have been some early complications (**Table 3**). Clinical results show a tendency for good and excellent clinical results in early and mid-term follow-up, but in time patients complain about toe position and pain in the tip of the toe with standard shoes. Patient satisfaction in 134 toes is shown in **Table 4**. Because of this incomplete satisfaction and pain in relation to the tip of the toes, we are evaluating the use of a shorter screw, which is introduced through the distal phalanx up to the middle phalanx, thereby not including the distal phalanx in the final fixation (**Table 4**).

SUMMARY

Treatment of rigid claw toe is still subject to discussion and evolution. Arthrodesis or arthroplasty of the PIPJ is apparently the most reliable procedure. K wire seems be the most reliable way to solve this clinical issue, but different implants specifically created to treat PIPJ deformities are being developed, and still have to be tested clinically. The use of screws to fix the PIPJ is a valid alternative, although some problems remain to be solved, specifically pain in relation to the tip of the screw. Longer follow-up studies are needed to increase our knowledge of the treatment of this specific deformity.

REFERENCES

1. Pastrana García F, Olivares Gutiérrez J, Bárcena Jiménez LR, et al. Tratamiento de la deformidad en garra de los dedos menores del pie. Acta Ortop Mex 2008;22(3):189–94 [in Spanish].
2. Schrier J, Louwerens JW, Verheyen C. Opinions on lesser toe deformities among Dutch othopaedic departments. Foot Ankle Int 2007;28(12):1265–70.
3. Ellington JK. Hammertoes and clawtoes: proximal interphalangeal joint correction. Foot Ankle Clin 2011;6(4):547–58.
4. Kwon J. The use of flexor to extensor transfers for the correction of the flexible hammer toe deformity. Foot Ankle Clin 2011;16:573–82.
5. Soule R. Operation for the correction of hammertoe. NY Med J 1910;41(13): 649–50.
6. Young C. An operation for the correction of hammertoe and claw-toe. J Bone Joint Surg 1938;20(3):715–9.
7. Du Vries HL. Dislocation of the toe. JAMA 1956;160:728.

8. Pichney G, Derner R, Lauf E. Digital "V" arthrodesis. J Foot Ankle Surg 1993; 32(5):473–9.
9. Miller JM, Blacklidge DK, Ferdowsian V, et al. Chevron arthrodesis of the interphalangeal joint for hammertoe correction. J Foot Ankle Surg 2010;49:194–6.
10. Coughlin MJ, Dorris J, Polk E. Operative repair of the fixed hammertoe deformity. Foot Ankle Int 2000;21(2):94–104.
11. Lehman DE, Smith RW. Treatment of symptomatic hammertoe with a proximal interphalangeal joint arthrodesis. Foot Ankle Int 1995;16(9):535–41.
12. Alvine FG, Garvin KL. Peg and dowel fusion of the proximal interphalangeal joint. Foot Ankle 1980;1(2):90–4.
13. Jones PC, Robinette J, Hahn PJ. A new technique for cylindrical peg-in-hole arthrodesis of the interphalangeal joint. J Foot Ankle Surg 2002;41(6):414–6.
14. Edwards WH, Beischer AD. Interphalangeal joint arthrodesis of the lesser toes. Foot Ankle Clin 2002;7:43–8.
15. Creighton RE, Blustein SM. Buried Kirschner wire fixation in digital fusion. J Foot Ankle Surg 1995;34:567–70.
16. Weil LS Jr. Hammertoe arthrodesis using conical reamers and internal pin fixation. J Foot Ankle Surg 1999;38(5):370–1.
17. Konkel KF, Menger AG, Retzlaff SA. Hammer toe correction using an absorbable intramedullary pin. Foot Ankle Int 2007;28(8):916–20.
18. Pietrzak WS, Lessek TP, Perns SV. A bioabsorbable fixation implant for use in proximal interphalangeal joint (hammer toe) arthrodesis: biomechanical testing in a synthetic bone substrate. J Foot Ankle Surg 2006;45(5):288–94.
19. Lane GD. Lesser digital fusion with a cannulated screw. J Foot Ankle Surg 2005; 44:172–94.
20. Caterini R, Farsetti P, Tarantino U, et al. Arthrodesis of the toe joints with an intramedullary cannulated screw for correction of hammertoe deformity. Foot Ankle Int 2004;25(4):256–61.
21. Roukis TS. A 1-piece shape-metal nitinol intramedullary internal fixation device for arthrodesis of the proximal interphalangeal joint in neuropathic patients with diabetes. Foot Ankle Spec 2009;2(3):130–4.
22. Bourke G. Trim-it spin pin: a new absorbable device for the treatment of claw and hammer toes by proximal interphalangeal joint fusion. Tech. Foot Ankle Surg 2009;8(3):139–45.

Osteotomy Considerations in Hallux Valgus Treatment

Improving the Correction Power

Emilio Wagner, MD*, Cristian Ortiz, MD

KEYWORDS

- Hallux valgus • Osteotomy • Correction power • Biomechanical evaluation
- Medial plates • Rotational scarf • Chevron • Proximal opening wedge
- Proximal closing wedge

KEY POINTS

- Osteotomies for hallux valgus treatment should be chosen depending on the preoperative deformity and the correction capacity of that particular osteotomy.
- To improve the correction power of a displacement osteotomy we can add rotation. Inversely to improve the power of a rotational osteotomy displacement should be added.
- Multiple points of fixation should be preferred for diaphyseal osteotomies; medial fixation should be preferred for proximal osteotomies.

INTRODUCTION

Many different treatment alternatives exist for hallux valgus surgery. Because none has been shown to be more effective than any other, more than 200 different surgeries have been designed. Osteotomies have been recommended for hallux valgus surgery for the last 2 decades, with good success rates and reliability over time.[1] The recurrence rate of the deformity depends on the preoperative deformity and also on the postoperative sesamoid reduction quality, being higher if the hallux valgus angle is greater than 37° to 40°, and if there is an incomplete reduction of the sesamoids after surgery.[2–4] For this reason, the correcting power for each procedure (ie, the intermetatarsal angle that an osteotomy can correct) should be known so that the best surgical procedure can be selected for every patient. In general, distal osteotomies are less powerful and are preferred for mild deformities. Proximal osteotomies are powerful and able to correct large intermetatarsal angles; they are the general choice for severe deformities.[5]

Author disclosures: The authors have no financial affiliations to disclose.

Clinica Alemana, Departamento de Traumatologia y Ortopedia, Vitacura 5951, Santiago, Chile

* Corresponding author.

E-mail address: emiliowagner@gmail.com

When correcting a hallux valgus deformity, the technique chosen should depend on the deformity to be corrected and the individual correction power a particular technique possesses. Although the classic intermetatarsal angle value is less than 9°, when correcting an hallux valgus deformity, there are individual variations in the angular measurements and not every hallux valgus is the same. Clinicians should try to achieve the best alignment and correction for each patient. In hallux valgus, the deformity comes from a medial deviation of the metatarsal bone, in which the sesamoids mark the original position where the metatarsal head was located.[6] The ideal position for the metatarsal head should be to lie on top of the sesamoid complex. An incomplete postoperative reduction of the sesamoids constitutes a risk factor for recurrence of the deformity.[4] Because of this, we currently use a new angular measurement to choose our osteotomy to correct the intermetatarsal angle, known as the angle to be corrected. This angle is obtained by drawing a line through the first metatarsal axis and then drawing a second line from the same starting point on the base of the first metatarsal but going distally through the middle of the sesamoid complex. This angle represents the number of degrees the metatarsal must be moved to center the head over the sesamoids.[7] After defining the correction power of each technique, the proper surgical procedure can be chosen, and this allows us to propose an algorithm of treatment. In this way, we have defined a surgical protocol in which, for angles to be corrected between 0° and 5°, we use the chevron osteotomy; for angular corrections between 5° and 9°, we suggest the rotational scarf osteotomy; and for angular corrections of more than 10°, we prefer a proximal osteotomy called POSCOW (proximal oblique closing wedge osteotomy).[7,8]

In an observational study performed in the United States regarding the preferred surgical techniques of academic foot and ankle surgeons, the chevron was the most common technique chosen for mild deformities in 87%, and the preferred techniques for severe deformities were first metatarsophalangeal arthrodesis (26%), cuneometatarsal arthrodesis (24%), Ludloff (24%), and proximal metatarsal osteotomies (24%).[9,10] This article discusses strategies and osteotomy considerations to improve the correction power of chevron, Ludloff, scarf, and proximal osteotomies for hallux valgus correction.

OSTEOTOMY OPTIONS
Chevron Osteotomy

Chevron osteotomies are inherently displacement osteotomies and, as such, they are limited by the width of the metatarsal bone. Five millimeters of lateral displacement for this osteotomy has traditionally been performed, and it is well known that it corrects 1° of intermetatarsal angle (IMA) per millimeter of lateral displacement. Biomechanical studies have shown that a 60° chevron osteotomy fails by rotation of the distal fragment in relation to the proximal fragment.[11] Increasing the angle between the arms of the osteotomy has been suggested as a way to increase compressive forces between the fragments, and therefore increase mechanical bonding.[12] The 90° chevron is currently our choice when performing a chevron osteotomy for mild deformities when the angle to be corrected is 5° or less. Another advantage of this modification is that it gives more room for fixation, our current preference being a 2.0 minifragment screw. Although no study has shown superiority between K wires or screws when fixing chevron osteotomies, we prefer to use fixation devices that do not need to be removed.

Modifications to increase the correction power refer to displacement maximization. Displacements up to 60% have been reported, with a 2-year follow-up with excellent results.[13] In these cases, only K wires can be used for fixation, preferably 2 to control rotation, and this has to be considered regarding the need for removal.

Diaphyseal Osteotomies

Diaphyseal osteotomies are either displacement or rotational osteotomies. Displacement osteotomies are limited, as are distal osteotomies, by the width of the bone. They can be displaced safely up to 5 mm, which limits their correction power, and they do not alter the distal metatarsal articular angle because they do not impose any rotation on the metatarsal bone. However, rotational or angular osteotomies do not have a width limitation, and theoretically have more correction power. They do alter the distal metatarsal articular angle because they impose some rotation to the metatarsal bone, and this is their most important limitation in their correction power.[14] The most well-known diaphyseal rotational or angular osteotomy is the Ludloff osteotomy.

Ludloff Osteotomy

This osteotomy was originally an oblique mid-diaphyseal osteotomy that started dorsally 1.5 cm distal to the metatarsocuneiform joint and progressed distally and plantarly, exiting proximal to the sesamoid complex.[15] It was later modified to achieve the longest osteotomy possible, starting as proximal to the tarsometatarsal joint as possible, with the lowest inclination possible, and ending just proximal to the sesamoid complex.[16] Another important consideration when rotating the osteotomy was that the closer the pivot point to the tarsometatarsal joint, the greater the correction achieved, and this can be understood using realignment concepts, which state that the closer to the center of rotation of angulation a deformity is corrected, the better the correction (with less translation) is achieved. Good intermediate-term results have been published regarding the modified Ludloff osteotomy, for 111 feet with an improvement of 35 points in the American Orthopaedic Foot and Ankle Score (AOFAS), with good angular improvements, and only 2.2 mm of shortening without dorsiflexion malunion.[17]

Efforts to further improve the correction power of this osteotomy have tried to increase the rotation, which therefore decreases the contact area and the intrinsic stability. Different modifications have been made to improve its fixation, namely K wires and plates.[18] Although no biomechanical study has evaluated the use of plates for diaphyseal osteotomies, dorsally and medially applied plates have been used for proximal osteotomies and have been shown to have an improved fixation,[19–21] and consequently it can be assumed that medially applied plates also improve diaphyseal osteotomy stiffness.

Scarf Osteotomy

The most well-known diaphyseal displacement osteotomy is the scarf osteotomy, which has been well described in the literature.[22,23] Its major theoretic advantage compared with a distal chevron osteotomy is a bigger area of bone contact (270 mm^2 compared with 116 mm^2 for the chevron[24]), which allows a greater displacement, therefore achieving a better correction of the deformity. It can correct up to 6° of intermetatarsal angle, limited by the width of the metatarsal bone.[25] Modifications such as short straight osteotomy arms instead of a 60° inclination apparently reduces the risk of troughing that has been reported in up to 35% of cases.[23] Regarding fixation, a 2-point fixation has traditionally been recommended, using Barouk screws, cannulated screws, or minifragment screws.[26] Based on our failures, a 3-point fixation achieves a larger area of contact between the fragments and therefore should decrease postoperative loss of correction. Failures have been seen with rotation of both fragments in relation to one of the screws, and therefore having an additional point of fixation should decrease the risk of correction failure. Structural failures are most commonly seen at the most proximal fixation site, that is, the proximal screw where the osteotomy runs longitudinally from plantar proximal to distal dorsal. Biomechanical studies have shown that the scarf osteotomy causes significant changes in stiffness and cortical bone strains at the proximal apex where a critical weakening is produced.[11] To avoid this type of failure, care must be taken to leave the dorsal shelf of bone as thick as possible at the proximal apex of the osteotomy.

Modifications to improve its correction power include increasing the lateral displacement, or adding rotation. Up to 7° of correction have been reported on the IMA angle to achieve more displacement, but without achieving a statistically significant difference compared with the chevron osteotomy.[27] When increasing displacement, the contact area decreases proportionally, and so care has to be taken when fixing it because failure risk and troughing may increase. Maximal displacements have been described in the literature, but with no clinical results to date, in which the medial cortex of the distal fragment of the metatarsal bone lines up with the lateral cortex of the proximal fragment, and an inside-out plating is performed to fix it.[28] The other modification described consists of adding rotation to this displacement osteotomy, which has been called the rotational scarf.

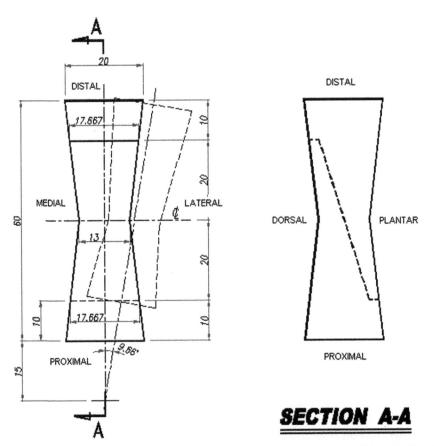

Fig. 1. Geometric model to estimate the maximum correction capacity of the rotational scarf osteotomy keeping bone contact in 50%. Section A-A shows a medial view of the osteotomy.

Rotational Scarf

To improve the correction power of the scarf osteotomy, rotation was added to it, using 2 of the more commonly used concepts in osteotomy execution: displacement and rotation. Described in 1992, the rotational scarf uses rotation in relation to the most proximal lateral aspect of the metatarsal bone, keeping the general shape of the scarf osteotomy, thus maintaining a broad bone contact between the fragments. In this way, better angular corrections with more than 50% of lateralization of the distal fragment can be achieved, keeping at least 50% of bone contact.[29] Recent clinical articles suggest that the rotational scarf decreases the risk of troughing[30] and the need for an Akin osteotomy,[31] although there is no evidence in the literature to prove it (the rotation imposed on the scarf osteotomy differs between studies).

The rotational scarf osteotomy can achieve geometrical correction through a proximal center of rotation, and has the power to correct up to 9° of intermetatarsal angle, maintaining bone contact in 50%.[7] The rotational scarf osteotomy with proximal center of rotation has been our choice for hallux valgus deformities during the last 5 years for patients with angles to be corrected between 5° and 9°. A geometric model was developed to study its correction power keeping bone contact in 50%, and its maximum correction power was calculated to be 9° (**Fig. 1**). We currently prefer 3 points of fixation (ie, 3 screws) because this theoretically should decrease the failure rate that we have seen when fixing the osteotomy with just 2 screws. The proximal aspect of the longitudinal osteotomy ends in a plantar situation, trying to leave a thick dorsal shelf of bone to reduce the risk of postoperative fracture, because this is the weakest point of the osteotomy (as mentioned earlier).

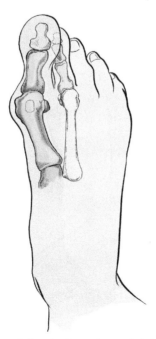

Fig. 2. A moderate hallux valgus deformity. Note the medial deviation of the first metatarsal and the subluxated sesamoid bones.

Surgical Technique

A medial longitudinal incision over the first metatarsophalangeal joint is performed (**Fig. 2**). An inverted-L capsulotomy is performed, exposing the metatarsal bone. The first metatarsal is exposed and dissected subperiosteally, leaving the lateral and plantar distal area intact to preserve circulation. A diaphyseal osteotomy is then performed, starting from plantar proximal to distal dorsal, with 2 arms oriented 90° to the main osteotomy line exiting through the plantar and dorsal cortex respectively (**Fig. 3**). The osteotomy is made as long as possible, normally measuring 4 cm in length. A translation and rotation around a proximally situated center of rotation is then performed, leaving approximately two-thirds of the width of the bone in contact proximally and one-third in contact between the 2 fragments distally, which corresponds approximately with 4 mm of displacement proximally and 11 mm of displacement distally (**Fig. 4**). This amount of displacement, because it is unequal in both bone ends, produces a lateral displacement and a rotation of the distal fragment, achieving a correction of approximately 8° to 9° of intermetatarsal angle. Because of small intraoperative changes caused by the internal fixation and because of postoperative bone remodeling, we have observed that a higher displacement is needed to achieve an adequate correction, and we currently displace distally almost 90% of the width of the metatarsal head, and proximally 30% of the width of the metatarsal base. Both fragments are held temporarily with a K wire and a bone clamp and fixed with 3 2.0-mm screws. We use three 2.0-mm screws from the compact foot set (Synthes, Switzerland), from the dorsal to the plantar aspect of the bone, unevenly spaced from proximal to distal. This disposition is used because of the larger area of bone contact obtained when using 3 screws and the increased theoretic resistance to torque when having screws at uneven distances. The overhanging bone is resected, and a traditional closure of the periosteum and capsule is performed (**Fig. 5**). Depending on the metatarsophalangeal balance after the metatarsal correction, a decision is made regarding the need to perform an Akin osteotomy. The subcutaneous and skin layers are closed with reabsorbable sutures. A postoperative dressing is applied, and a postoperative shoe is used. See **Figs. 6** and **7** for preoperative and postoperative radiographs from a clinical example.

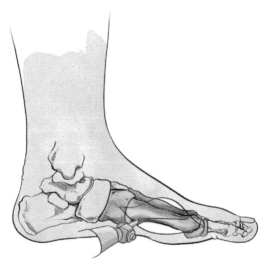

Fig. 3. Medial view of rotational scarf osteotomy. Note the diaphyseal osteotomy performed as long as possible, starting from distal dorsal to plantar proximal, with 2 arms oriented 90° to the main osteotomy line exiting through the plantar and dorsal cortex.

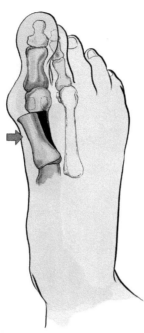

Fig. 4. The distal and proximal displacement of the rotational scarf osteotomy, leaving a medial overhanging bone that is resected later (*arrow*). The distal displacement is as great as possible, reaching 90% of the width of the bone. The proximal displacement is approximately 30% of the width of the bone, thereby achieving a rotational effect.

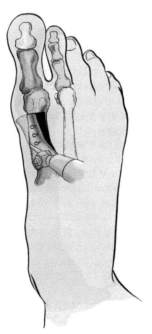

Fig. 5. Fixation of the osteotomy has already been performed with three 2.0-mm screws. The medial overhanging bone is resected. The total displacement is represented by the black area of the metatarsal bone.

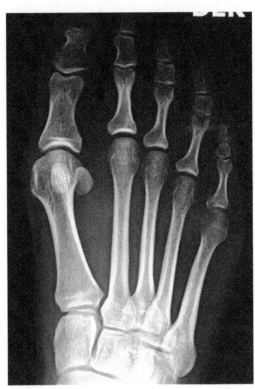

Fig. 6. Preoperative radiograph of a patient with a moderate hallux valgus deformity. Note the mild subluxation of the sesamoid complex.

RESULTS

Rotational scarf osteotomy results have been published recently, but there are technical differences within the same technique. In 2011, Murawski[30] showed a rotational scarf but with a center of rotation of angulation near the middle of the metatarsal bone, as they rotate both the distal and the proximal ends. This center of rotation allows correction of the intermetatarsal angle with alteration of the distal metatarsal articular angle, and the investigators did not take advantage of any lateral displacement of the plantar fragment. Although theoretically it has a similar center of rotation as the Mau osteotomy, and therefore its potential to correct intermetatarsal angle could be low, the results showed a large correction power, with 10° of intermetatarsal angle improvement (before surgery 18°, range 9°–23°; after surgery 8°, range 6°–12°). A later article also dealt with rotational scarf osteotomies, but using a proximal center of rotation with more displacement distally than proximally.[31] In that article, 34 feet were evaluated, operated on with the rotational scarf osteotomy, and minimum follow-up was 12 months (average 26.4 months). There was a 94% satisfaction rate, the hallux valgus angle improved from 34.6° to 14.9°, and the intermetatarsal angle improved from 15.8° to 7.2°.

In the last 5 years we have performed more than 500 rotational scarf osteotomies with a proximal center of rotation, almost always with good to excellent results. We have followed a small series of 18 patients since 2007; 28 feet, all treated with a rotational scarf osteotomy. Average age was 49.8 years, mean follow-up was 54 months. The satisfaction rate was 94.5%, with a mean AOFAS score of 97.6 points. The

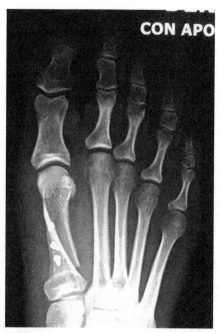

Fig. 7. Postoperative radiograph of the patient shown in **Fig. 6**. Note the maximal displacement achieved distally. Three screws are used to fix the osteotomy. Excellent correction can be achieved and no additional correction is needed.

intermetatarsal angle improvement was 7.4° (before surgery 14.8°, range 8.7°–16.7°; after surgery 7.4°, range 3.4°–11.5°). The metatarsophalangeal angle improved 11.8° (before surgery 23.7°, range 14°–27.5°; after surgery 11.9°, range 1.7°–16.6°). An Akin was needed in 4 feet (14%). In these series, we have only 1 case with persistent metatarsalgia, which was in the unsatisfied patient.

Proximal Osteotomies

Proximal osteotomies are either displacement osteotomies, like the proximal chevron osteotomy in which correction is achieved through lateral displacement, or angular osteotomies such as the proximal crescentic osteotomy, in which rotation is performed to achieve correction of the intermetatarsal angle. For distal and diaphyseal osteotomies, the correction power of proximal displacement osteotomies are limited by the width of the bone, which, in the base of the first metatarsal, corresponds with approximately 20 mm, and therefore 10 mm of displacement is considered the maximum possible translation to keep bone contact in 50%. These osteotomies correct 1° of intermetatarsal angle per millimeter of lateral translation, and therefore they are not powerful techniques.

For severe deformities, angular osteotomies have been recommended because they achieve more correction.[14] Angular osteotomies achieve correction through rotation in relation to a proximal center of rotation, which immediately gives them an increased correction power, at the same time increasing the distal metatarsal articular angle. Some examples of angular osteotomies are the proximal crescentic osteotomy, proximal opening wedge osteotomy, and proximal closing wedge osteotomy. A combined osteotomy (POSCOW) has also been presented that uses displacement and rotation, thereby using both concepts of osteotomy correction and requiring less alteration of the distal metatarsal articular angle.

Proximal Chevron Osteotomy

This osteotomy was first described by Sammarco.[32] It consists mainly of a lateral displacement osteotomy, and is limited by the width of the bone, which gives it a mild correction power[14] of approximately 1° of intermetatarsal angle corrected per millimeter of lateral displacement. It is more stable than a proximal crescentic osteotomy because of its geometry, thereby avoiding dorsiflexion malunion of the first metatarsal or shortening of the bone.[33]

Improvements in its correction power regarding technique and fixation have been achieved. Regarding technique, besides lateral displacement, some angular correction has been added, with impaction of the lateral side of the osteotomy achieving good correction power, with 20° of hallux valgus correction and 9.5° of intermetatarsal angle correction.[33] Improving fixation to reliably preserve the correction has also been attempted. Medial locking plates have been described as having excellent results, achieving 16° of hallux valgus improvement and 7.6° of intermetatarsal angle improvement, with an average AOFAS score of 94 points,[21] with no transfer lesion after surgery.

Proximal Crescentic Osteotomy

This osteotomy was popularized by Mann.[34] Because it uses a crescentic saw blade, it achieves an excellent correction of the intermetatarsal angle through angular rotation at the base of the metatarsal bone. Because it is a mainly vertical osteotomy, it is less stable than the proximal chevron, and therefore it needs strong fixation to be stable. Good results have been shown using fixation with just a screw and a K wire, with a hallux valgus angle correction of 22° and an intermetatarsal angle correction of 9°, with just 17% of dorsiflexion malunion, which is less than was originally described.[33] Efforts to improve its fixation to avoid malunion have been reported, such as using dorsal plates, which have been shown in cadaveric studies to produce a 100% improvement in the resistance to failure of the construct.[35] Clinical studies reporting dorsal plates have shown excellent satisfaction rates, with corrections of 17.9° of hallux valgus angle and 6.6° of intermetatarsal angle improvement.[36] Another option to avoid dorsiflexion malunion is to incorporate into the osteotomy a plantar flexion position of the metatarsal bone, rotating it plantarly after performing the osteotomy. However, although theoretically attractive, no real advantage in terms of arch height improvement or increased first metatarsal declination angle has been shown with this modification.[37]

Proximal Opening Wedge Osteotomy

This was first described in 1923 but instability and concerns about nonunion made it unpopular.[5] This osteotomy mainly corrects the intermetatarsal angle through lateral rotation of the metatarsal bone with the addition of medial wedges of different sizes. It can lengthen the bone and increase the distal metatarsal articular angle because the correction is achieved through angular correction without any displacement. It has increased in popularity in the last few years, with the advent of new plating techniques that use locking plates with fixed opening wedge sizes. Proximal opening wedge osteotomies are stable osteotomies in which the lateral cortex should not be violated, but a medially placed locking plate construct can perform equally well regarding stiffness, even compared with Ludloff constructs, at least in initial cyclic loading in a cadaveric study.[38] Clinical studies show excellent results, with hallux valgus angle improvements of 14.7° and intermetatarsal angle improvement of 6.4°. The mean increase in metatarsal length was 2.3 mm, which cannot be associated with any symptom related to tightening of soft tissues like decreased metatarsophalangeal range of motion[39] or predisposition to jamming of the metatarsophalangeal joint.[40]

Efforts to improve its correction power have focused on increasing the medial wedge without violating the integrity of the lateral cortex. A linear relation seems to exist between the size of the medial wedge and the correction achieved, although it plateaus using the 6-mm opening wedge plate.[39] Concern still remains regarding the possible effect on metatarsophalangeal pressure and its limit in correction power because, although reported to correct 3° per millimeter of opening wedge, the average improvement in intermetatarsal angle ranges from 6° to 10°.[39–41]

Proximal Closing Wedge Osteotomy

Compared with an opening wedge osteotomy, the main difference of this osteotomy is that it shortens the metatarsal bone, and therefore there is no concern regarding changes in intraarticular pressure or decreased range of motion, but it also alters the distal metatarsal articular angle because all the angular correction is achieved through the resected wedge. Good to excellent results in up to 85% of patients have been reported with basilar closing wedge osteotomies, but concern exists regarding complications such as dorsiflexion malunion and first metatarsal shortening and subsequent transfer metatarsalgia.[5] To overcome these risks, efforts have been made to increase fixation strength using plates. Results from more than 70 hallux valgus feet operated on with a first metatarsal closing wedge osteotomy fixed with dorsal minifragment plates were recently reported.[42] The average hallux valgus angle improvement was 20° and

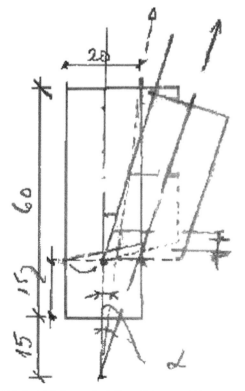

Fig. 8. Geometric model used for calculating the correction power of the POSCOW osteotomy.

the intermetatarsal angle improvement was 8.8°. The absolute first metatarsal shortening was only 2.2 mm, and sagittal first metatarsal alignment showed just 1.3° of dorsiflexion. These results probably indicate a refined surgical technique and the advantages of using strong fixation to ensure good postoperative alignment.

Combined Osteotomy: POSCOW Osteotomy

To combine the advantages of proximal displacement osteotomies (which maintain metatarsal length and do not alter the distal metatarsal articular angle) and the correction power of angular osteotomies (which can correct as many degrees as wanted, depending on the rotation imposed on the metatarsal), a modification of a closing wedge technique was designed and named POSCOW.[8] This technique has been our choice for many years, and we recommend it for hallux valgus deformities in which the angle to be corrected is more than 10°. Our first cases were fixed with dorsal minifragment plates, and over the years, we changed to minifragment locked medial plates. Using medial fixation improves the stiffness of the construct over dorsal plates by 158% if using titanium locked plates and 228% when using steel nonlocked plates

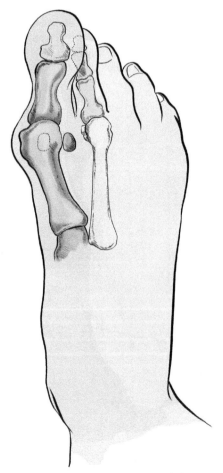

Fig. 9. A severe hallux valgus deformity. Note the medial deviation of the first metatarsal and the complete dislocation of the sesamoid bones.

(personal investigation, not published). A geometric model was designed to study its correction power and how to determine the size of the resected wedge and the lateral displacement (**Fig. 8**). It was determined that a lateral proximal displacement of 5 mm would correct 4° of intermetatarsal angle and that, to correct 1° of additional interme-tatarsal angle, a bone wedge with a lateral base of 0.4 mm had to be resected. because the osteotomy is performed perpendicular in both planes (transverse and sagittal) to the metatarsal bone, its plane is oblique in relation to the second metatarsal bone, going proximal medial to lateral distal. Thus, with the lateral displacement, a slight lengthening of the bone is achieved. This lengthening was calculated to be 1.3 mm for an IMA angle of 15°, and 1.8 mm for an angle of 20°. This lengthening partially compensates for the expected shortening any closing wedge osteotomy produces.

Surgical Technique

A medial longitudinal incision over the first metatarsophalangeal joint is performed (**Fig. 9**). An inverted-L capsulotomy is performed, exposing the metatarsal bone. The first metatarsal is exposed and dissected subperiosteally, leaving the lateral and plantar distal area intact to preserve circulation. A careful resection of the bunion is performed following the medial cortex of the metatarsal bone. Then a proximal metatarsal osteotomy is performed, with a straight cut from the dorsal to the plantar aspect of the metatarsal bone 15 mm distal to the base of the bone and perpendicular to the long axis of the metatarsal bone (**Fig. 10**). Depending on the angular correction needed, a laterally based wedge of bone is removed from the proximal aspect of the distal fragment, as determined in the preoperative planning. A lateral displacement of 5 mm is performed, moving the base of the metatarsal bone laterally (**Fig. 11**).

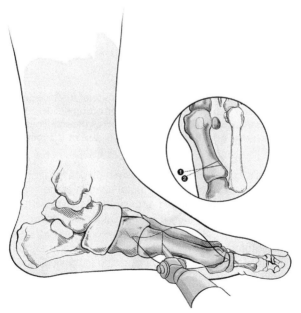

Fig. 10. A proximal metatarsal osteotomy, with a straight cut from the dorsal to the plantar aspect of the metatarsal bone 15 mm distal to the base of the bone and perpendicular to the long axis of the metatarsal bone. In the inset figure, the lateral closing wedge of bone is drawn. It is performed with 2 straight divergent cuts (1 and 2) from the medial aspect of the metatarsal bone.

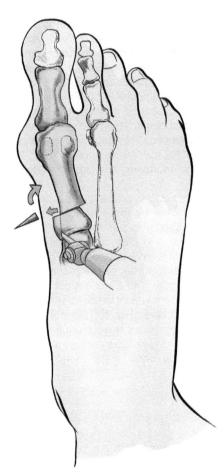

Fig. 11. After removing the lateral closing wedge, a lateral displacement of 5 mm of the distal fragment is performed, achieving the angular correction needed. This position is fixed temporarily by two 1.6-mm K wires. Note the reduction of the sesamoid complex under the metatarsal head. The overhanging bone of the medial base of the metatarsal is resected.

Fluoroscopic control is taken to ensure parallelism between the first and second metatarsals and adequate reduction of the metatarsal head over the sesamoids. The fixation is performed with a medially placed angular stable plate with 2 locking screws distally and 2 locked screws proximally (**Fig. 12**). Depending on the metatarsophalangeal balance after the metatarsal correction, a decision is made regarding the need to perform an Akin osteotomy. The capsule, subcutaneous, and skin layers are closed with reabsorbable sutures. A postoperative dressing is applied, and a postoperative shoe is used. A clinical example is shown in **Fig. 13**.

RESULTS

Our results from 56 feet (mean age 55 years, follow-up of 35 months) show a satisfaction rate of 87%. The average improvement was 24° for the hallux valgus angle and 11° for the intermetatarsal angle. The mean first metatarsal shortening was 1.5 mm. Deformity recurrence requiring revision was observed in 7% of the cases, most commonly

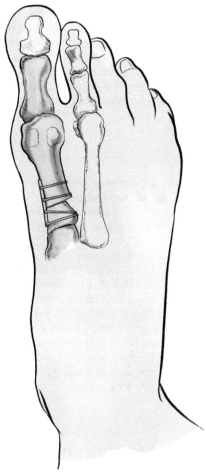

Fig. 12. The fixation is performed with a medially placed angular stable plate with 2 locking screws distally and 2 locked screws proximally.

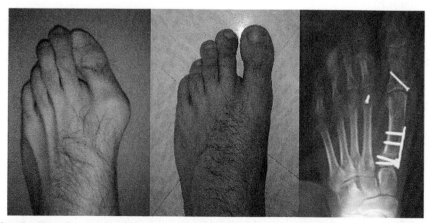

Fig. 13. Clinical example of a severe hallux valgus deformity, with preoperative and postoperative views and the postoperative radiograph.

solved with the addition of a distal chevron osteotomy. We had 1 nonunion that required revision and 1 failed fixation that resolved with immobilization in a cam walker. Transfer metatarsalgia was observed in 3.5% of the cases. Most of the complications occurred in the first year of use of this osteotomy, because the learning curve included the use of both displacement and rotation, and the optimization of the fixation method. We observed less shortening than expected, and we think that performing the osteotomy in an oblique fashion compensates for the shortening caused by the closing wedge.

SUMMARY

Efforts are currently being made to improve results in hallux valgus treatment. Different studies to design procedures that are more stable and efficient to correct deformities are underway, and new techniques will be presented in the following years. Better fixation devices will offer reliability in corrections, and hopefully will allow faster rehabilitation with fewer restrictions.

Understanding the concept of correction power is important when deciding which technique to use. The origin of hallux valgus is not known, but evidence exists to assume that a correct skeletal and soft tissue balance is important to prevent recurrence and obtain good function. We think that a correct metatarsophalangeal reduction, in which the final position of the hallux is defined mainly by the skeletal alignment and not soft tissues, will dictate the final result. Pushing the metatarsal bone over the sesamoids and not moving the sesamoids under the metatarsal head is a new concept and it may allow better results for our patients. It is hoped that understanding of biomechanics will continue to evolve, and radiological measurements and corrections will produce better functional results for patients.

REFERENCES

1. Trnka HJ. Osteotomies for hallux valgus correction. Foot Ankle Clin North Am 2005;10:15–33.
2. Deenik AR, de Visser E, Louwerens JW, et al. Hallux valgus angle as a main predictor for correction of hallux valgus. BMC Musculoskelet Disord 2008; 15(9):70.
3. Okuda R, Kinoshita M, Yasuda T, et al. Hallux valgus angle as a predictor of recurrence following proximal metatarsal osteotomy. J Orthop Sci 2011;16(6): 760–4.
4. Okuda R, Kinoshita M, Yasuda T, et al. Postoperative incomplete reduction of the sesamoids as a risk factor for recurrence of hallux valgus. J Bone Joint Surg Am 2009;91(7):1637–45.
5. Easley ME, Trnka HJ. Current concepts review: hallux valgus part II: operative treatment. Foot Ankle Int 2007;28(6):748–58.
6. Tanaka Y, Takakura Y. Precise anatomic configuration changes in the first ray of the hallux valgus foot. Foot Ankle Int 2000;21:651–6.
7. Wagner E, Ortiz C, Keller A. Modified diaphyseal osteotomy with a proximal center of rotation for moderate to severe hallux valgus. Tech Foot Ankle Surg 2007;6(2):113–7.
8. Wagner E, Ortiz C, Keller A. Proximal oblique slide closing wedge metatarsal osteotomy with plate fixation for severe hallux valgus deformities. Tech Foot Ankle Surg 2007;6(4):270–4, 2007.

9. Pinney S, Song K, Chou L. Surgical treatment of mild hallux valgus deformity: the state of practice among academic foot and ankle surgeons. Foot Ankle Int 2006; 27(11):970–3.

10. Pinney SJ, Song KR, Chou LB. Surgical treatment of severe hallux valgus: the state of practice among academic foot and ankle surgeons. Foot Ankle Int 2006;27(12):1024–9.

11. Favre P, Farine M, Snedeker JG, et al. Biomechanical consequences of first metatarsal osteotomy in treating hallux valgus. Clin Biomech 2010;25:721–7.

12. Matzaroglou C, Bougas P, Panagiotopoulos E, et al. Ninety-degree chevron osteotomy for correction of hallux valgus deformity: clinical data and finite element analysis. Open Orthop J 2010;22(4):152–6.

13. Murawski DE, Beskin JL. Increased displacement maximizes the utility of the distal chevron osteotomy for hallux valgus correction. Foot Ankle Int 2008; 29(2):155–63.

14. Nyska M, Trnka HJ, Parks BG, et al. Proximal metatarsal osteotomies: a comparative geometric analysis conducted on sawbone models. Foot Ankle Int 2002;23: 938–45.

15. Bae S, Schon LC. Surgical strategies: Ludloff first metatarsal osteotomy. Foot Ankle Int 2007;28(1):137–44.

16. Beischer A, Ammon P, Corniou A, et al. Three-dimensional computer analysis of the modified Ludloff osteotomy. Foot Ankle Int 2005;26(8):627–32.

17. Trnka HJ, Hofstaetter SG, Easley ME. Intermediate-term results of the Ludloff osteotomy in one hundred and eleven feet. Surgical technique. J Bone Joint Surg Am 2009;91(S2):156–68.

18. Stamatis ED, Chatzikomminos IE, Karaoglanis GC. Locking plate as "medial buttress" for oblique osteotomy for hallux valgus. Foot Ankle Int 2010;31(10):920–2.

19. Scott AT, DeOrio JK, Montijo HE, et al. Biomechanical comparison of hallux valgus correction using the proximal chevron osteotomy fixed with a medial locking plate and the Ludloff osteotomy fixed with two screws. Clin Biomech 2010; 25(3):271–6.

20. Jones C, Coughlin M, Petersen W, et al. Mechanical comparison of two types of fixation for proximal first metatarsal crescentic osteotomy. Foot Ankle Int 2005; 26(5):371–4.

21. Gallentine JW, DeOrio JK, DeOrio MJ. Bunion surgery using locking-plate fixation of proximal metatarsal chevron osteotomies. Foot Ankle Int 2007;28(3):361–8.

22. Barouk LS. Scarf osteotomy for hallux valgus correction. Local anatomy, surgical technique, and combination with other forefoot procedures. Foot Ankle Clin 2000; 5(1):525–58.

23. Coetzee JC, Rippstein P. Surgical strategies: scarf osteotomy for hallux valgus. Foot Ankle Int 2007;28(4):529–35.

24. Vienne P, Favre P, Meyer D, et al. Comparative mechanical testing of different geometric designs of distal first metatarsal osteotomies. Foot Ankle Int 2007; 28(2):232–6.

25. Dereymaeker G. Scarf osteotomy for correction of hallux valgus. Surgical technique and results as compared to distal chevron osteotomy. Foot Ankle Clin 2000;5(3):513–24.

26. Gupta S, Fazal MA, Williams L. Minifragment screw fixation of the scarf osteotomy. Foot Ankle Int 2008;29(4):385–9.

27. Deenik A, van Mameren H, de Visser E, et al. Equivalent correction in scarf and chevron osteotomy in moderate and severe hallux valgus: a randomized controlled trial. Foot Ankle Int 2008;29(12):1209–15.

28. Bouaicha S, Moor BK, Bohnert L, et al. Fixation of maximal shift scarf osteotomy with inside-out plating: technique tip. Foot Ankle Int 2011;32(5):S567–9.
29. Duke HF. Rotational scarf (Z) osteotomy bunionectomy for correction of high inter-metatarsal angles. J Am Podiatr Med Assoc 1992;82(7):352–60.
30. Murawski CD, Egan CJ, Kennedy JG. A rotational scarf osteotomy decreases troughing when treating hallux valgus. Clin Orthop Relat Res 2011;469(3): 847–53.
31. Adam SP, Choung SC, Gu Y, et al. Outcomes after scarf osteotomy for treatment of adult hallux valgus deformity. Clin Orthop Relat Res 2011;469(3):854–9.
32. Sammarco GJ, Brainard B, Sammarco VJ. Bunion correction using proximal chevron osteotomy. Foot Ankle Int 1993;14(1):8–14.
33. Easley ME, Kiebzak GM, Hodges DW, et al. Prospective, randomized comparison of proximal crescentic and proximal chevron osteotomies for correction of hallux valgus deformity. Foot Ankle Int 1997;17(6):307–16.
34. Mann R, Rudicel S, Graves S. Repair of hallux valgus with a distal soft tissue procedure and proximal metatarsal osteotomy. A long-term follow-up. J Bone Joint Surg Am 1992;74(1):124–9.
35. Varner KE, Matt V, Alexander JW, et al. Screw versus plate fixation of proximal first metatarsal crescentic osteotomy. Foot Ankle Int 2009;30(2):142–9.
36. Yuen-hon Chow F, Lui TH, Kwok KW, et al. Plate fixation for crescentic metatarsal osteotomy in the treatment of hallux valgus: an eight-year followup study. Foot Ankle Int 2008;29(1):29–33.
37. Tanaka Y, Takakura Y, Kumai T, et al. Proximal spherical metatarsal osteotomy for the foot with severe hallux valgus. Foot Ankle Int 2008;29(10):1025–30.
38. Hofstaetter SG, Glisson RR, Alitz CJ, et al. Biomechanical comparison of screws and plates for hallux valgus opening-wedge and Ludloff osteotomies. Clin Biomech 2008;23(1):101–8.
39. Shurnas PS, Watson TS, Crislip TW. Proximal first metatarsal opening wedge osteotomy with a low profile plate. Foot Ankle Int 2009;30(9):865–72.
40. Saragas NP. Proximal opening-wedge osteotomy of the first metatarsal for hallux valgus using a low profile plate. Foot Ankle Int 2009;30(10):976–80.
41. Smith WB, Hyer CF, DeCarbo WT, et al. Opening wedge osteotomies for correction of hallux valgus: a review of wedge plate fixation. Foot Ankle Spec 2009;2: 277–82.
42. Day TD, Charlton TP, Thordarson DB. First metatarsal length change after basilar closing wedge osteotomy for hallux valgus. Foot Ankle Int 2011;32(5):513–8.

Index

Note: Page numbers of article titles are in **boldface** type.

Foot Ankle Clin N Am 17 (2012) 499–516
http://dx.doi.org/10.1016/S1083-7515(12)00080-0
1083-7515/12/$ – see front matter © 2012 Elsevier Inc. All rights reserved.

foot.theclinics.com



Moving?

Make sure your subscription moves with you!

To notify us of your new address, find your **Clinics Account Number** (located on your mailing label above your name), and contact customer service at:

Email: journalscustomerservice-usa@elsevier.com

800-654-2452 (subscribers in the U.S. & Canada)
314-447-8871 (subscribers outside of the U.S. & Canada)

Fax number: 314-447-8029

Elsevier Health Sciences Division
Subscription Customer Service
3251 Riverport Lane
Maryland Heights, MO 63043

*To ensure uninterrupted delivery of your subscription, please notify us at least 4 weeks in advance of move.

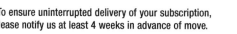

Printed and bound by CPI Group (UK) Ltd, Croydon, CR0 4YY

03/10/2024

01040436-0008